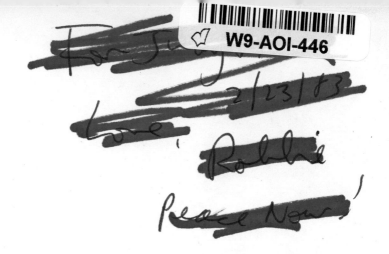

TO YOUR GOOD HEALTH!

A Practical Guide for Older Americans,
Their Families and Friends

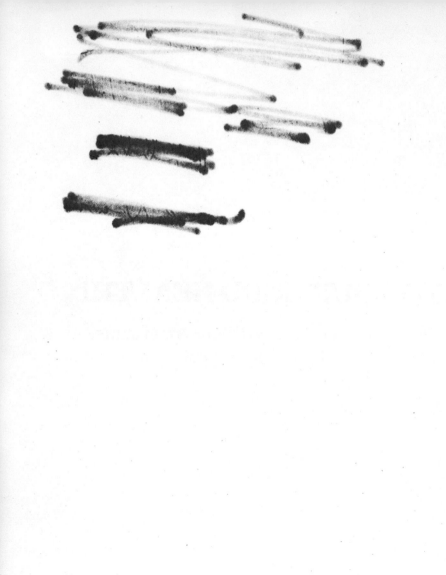

TO YOUR GOOD HEALTH!

A Practical Guide for Older Americans, Their Families and Friends
by Robert J. Skeist, R. N.

Foreword by Maggie Kuhn, with Contributions from Robert Butler, M. D. , Ken Dychtwald, Ph.D., and others.

Chicago Review Press

Cover design by Joseph Essex
Typography and Assembly by Accent Graphics,
Chicago, Illinois

Author's photo (back cover)
by Michael Kulczycki, Augustana Hospital

Library of Congress Cataloging in Publication Data
Skeist, Robert J. 1948-   To Your Good Health!
    1. Aged-care and hygiene.
  I. Butler, Robert N., joint author.
 II. Dychtwald, Ken, 1950- joint author.
III. Title.
RA777.6.S59   613'.0438   80-11173
ISBN 0-914090-83-6

**Published by: Chicago Review Press,
Chicago**

*Dedicated with love to my grandmother, Anna Geist,
and to the memory of my grandparents David Geist,
Bertha Skeist, and Samuel Skeist*

CONTENTS

Contents... vii

List of Contributors....................................... ix

Foreword/*Maggie Kuhn*.................................. xvii

Preface.. xxi

I: The Basics of Good Health

1. Exercise: Walking and the "Daily 21" 3

2. Eating for Health, Flavor and Economy................ 25

3. A Sense of Meaning, A Sense of Balance 51

4. Sleeping Without Pills 57

II: Twelve Common Problems and What to Do about Them

5. "Oh, My Aching Joints!" How to Cope with Arthritis.... 67

6. Caring for your Teeth, Gums and Dentures/
   Marsha Pike Palmer................................ 77

7. The Eyes Have It 89

8. "I Hear You!" Hearing Changes, Hearing Aids 97

9. Be Good to Your Feet/*Robert J. Skeist,
   Leonard Winston*....................................103

10. Be of Strong Heart!/*Susan Nick* 111

11. Controlling Diabetes...................................121

12. Up in Smoke 127

13. Cancer — Reducing Your Risk 131

14. Aches and Pains/*Susan Nick* 141

15. Safety Check List. 149

16. Surviving Vacations, Summer's Heat
    and Winter's Chill 153

III: Feelings

17. Changes in Women's Lives: Rose's Story/*Ruth Huang* ... 177

18. Sex at Any Age/*Barbara Giovannoni,
    Joseph Giovannoni* 185

19. Gray and Gay/*Richard Steinman* 199

20. Dealing with Losses/*Sanford Finkel* 203

21. Grieving: A Natural Part of Life/*Laurieann Chutis*. 221

22. Massage: It's Nice to be Kneaded/*Robert King* 231

23. Smooth to the Touch on Top 245

IV: Surviving the Medical System

24. Patients Have Rights! 251

25. Understanding Medical Language/*Leo Schlosberg* 267

26. Medications — They Should Help You,
    Not Hurt You 275

27. Paying the Bills: A Guide to Medicare,
    Supplemental Insurance and Medicaid/*J. Ram Ray*... 295

V: How Things Should Be

28. Changing the Medical System:
    An Interview with Robert Butler, M. D. 319

29. Building Support Groups: Sage and the Association
    for Humanistic Gerontology/*Ken Dychtwald*. 325

30. We Can Do It! An Interview with Maggie Kuhn 337

Chapters not otherwise credited are by Robert J. Skeist

LIST OF CONTRIBUTORS

Robert J. Skeist, R. N., is a graduate of the Ravenswood Hospital Medical Center School of Nursing (1975) and the Urban Preceptorship Program in Urban Health Care Delivery of the University of Illinois at the Medical Center, Department of Preventive Medicine (1977), where he developed an exercise program for older people. He has studied massage, meditation, and Tai Chi Ch'uan and taught modified versions of these health-promoting techniques to older people and professionals. As author of "Staying Healthy," a regular feature of Chicago's *Weekly Review*, and as Manager of the Seniors' Health Program of Augustana Hospital, he provides useful information on a wide range of health topics to thousands of senior citizens, their family members, and those who work with them. He lectures locally and nationally on aging and medication safety and serves as consultant to governmental, religious, and private social service agencies.

Mr. Skeist is a member of the American Nurses Association, the Association for Humanistic Gerontology, and the American Public Health Association. He has participated for a decade and a half in movements for social change, sings with the Yiddish folk group Der Driter Dor, and is active in the Gray Panthers.

Laurieann Chutis, M. S. W. , A. C. S. W. , holds a Bachelors Degree in Psychology and a Masters in Social Work from the University of Michigan. She is a graduate of the three-year training program of the Gestalt Institute of Chicago and has studied family therapy with Virginia Satir. She is Director of Consultation and Education Services at Ravenswood Hospital Community Mental Health Center, for which she received the 1976-77 Regional Award of the National Council of Community Mental Health Centers for outreach programs to the geriatric population. She has a private practice in individual, group, and sex therapy and is author of "Self Help Groups," a monograph of the National Council of Community Mental Health Centers, Inc.

Ken Dychtwald, Ph.D. , psychologist, is a pioneer in the holistic health and human development fields. He is presently President of the Association for Humanistic Gerontology, and was formerly Director of the Sage Project, the highly acclaimed holistic health center for elders in Berkeley, California.

In addition to lecturing and conducting seminars nationwide on bodymind development, holistic health and aging/longevity, he serves as a consultant to government, industry and media and is an adjunct instructor in psychology, gerontology and health related sciences at several universities.

His publications include *Bodymind* (JOVE 1978), *Millenium: Glimpses into the 21st Century* (with Dr. A. Villoldo, Teacher/St. Martins 1980), *Life Design* (forthcoming) and numerous articles in professional journals and popular magazines on health, aging/longevity, fitness, sports and human transformation.

Sanford I. Finkel, M. D., is coordinator of Health Services for the Elderly for the State of Illinois Department of Mental Health Region 2, is Assistant Professor of Clinical Psychiatry at Northwestern University Medical Center, and has a private practice in psychiatry. He received his Bachelor's and Medical degrees from the University of Michigan and was Chief of Geriatric Psychiatry at Michael Reese Hospital from 1968-76. He is Founder and President of the American Association for Geriatric Psychiatry and Co-Founder for the Society for Life Cycle Psychology in Aging.

Barbara Giovannoni holds a Bachelor of Arts degree in English Literature from Roosevelt University in Chicago and is working on a graduate degree in clinical psychology. She conducts resocialization groups in nursing homes.

Joseph Giovannoni, R. N. , M. A. , received his Masters Degree in Psychology from Roosevelt University 1977 and additional training at Loyola University Department of Psychiatry's Sexual Dysfunction Clinic. He is certified by the American Association of Sex Educators, Counsellors, and Therapists. He is an instructor of nursing at Augustana Hospital School of Nursing in Chicago, has a private practice in sexual dysfunction and marital counseling at Barkley Hospital in Chicago, and provides continuing education sessions for nursing home staff.

Dori Gordon will graduate in June 1980 with a Bachelor's of Science degree in Biocommunication from the University of Illinois Medical Center in Chicago. She is a freelance medical illustrator.

Ruth Huang, R. N. , graduated from the University of Michigan with a Bachelors of Fine Arts (1969), and from Grace Hospital School of Nursing in Detroit (1974). She received training in 1979 at the Sexual Dysfunction Clinic of Loyola University's School of Medicine, and will graduate in August 1980 from Rush University with an M. S. N. — a master's degree in psychiatric nursing. She is active in H. E. R. S. , a Chicago feminist health organization.

Robert King, who holds a Bachelor of Arts in Philosophy from Oglethorpe College in Atlanta

1970, is Illinois President of the American Massage and Therapy Association and Spa Director at Chicago's Ritz Carlton Hotel. He conducts workshops for hospital psychiatric staffs and patients on physical fitness and massage and has a private massage practice. He serves as consultant to the Seniors' Health Program of Augustana Hospital on massage techniques for older people.

Susan Nick, R. N., M. S. N., holds a Bachelors Degree in Nursing from City University of New York and a Masters Degree as a Medical/Surgical Clinical Specialist in Gerontological Nursing from Loyola University of Chicago 1979. She has worked on medical/surgical and neurological nursing units and has a special interest in stress and pain-reduction. She is Health Educator at the Seniors' Health Program of Augustana Health Hospital in Chicago.

Marsha Pike Palmer, R. D. H., M. A., holds a Bachelor of Science in Dental Hygiene from the University of Michigan (1970) and a Master of Arts in Curriculum Administration from De Paul University in Chicago (1979). She is Director of Dental Hygiene Education for the American Dental Association. She has nine years' experience in clinical dentistry and patient education and has developed a geriatric community education program for the Chicago Dental Hygiene Association.

J. Ram Ray is Editor/Executive Director of *Weekly Review*, a paper he founded in 1975 to provide news and features for older people in the Chicago area. He holds a B. A. in journalism and an M. A. in economics from Osmania University, Hyder-Abad, India, an M. A. in Communication Arts for the Department of Speech and Dramatic Art, University of Missouri 1974. He conducts workshops on media and aging and is a financial Consultant with *Discovery — 60*.

Leo Schlosberg is President of Infocorp, a computerized information retrieval business. He teaches courses on a social science view of medicine at De Paul University in Chicago. He has done technical writing in medicine. He holds a Bachelor's Degree in Psychology from the University of Chicago and graduated from the Urban Preceptorship Program in Urban Health Care Delivery of the University of Illinois at the Medical Center.

Richard Steinman, Ph.D., is Professor of Social Welfare at the University of Southern Maine. He conducts research and does writing on issues related to the elderly and to homosexuality.

Leonard Winston, D. P. M., graduated from the Illinois College of Podiatric Medicine 1961. He supervises podiatric students in foot care for older people, is chairman of the Speakers' Bureau of the Illinois Podiatric Society, and teaches at the Illinois

College of Podiatric Medicine and at Forkosh Hospital. Dr. Winston conducts seminars for joggers and
has a private practice in Chicago.

FOREWORD

Health is a basic human right. All of us need and want good health, but all too often we take it for granted until we lose it and try to get it back. Many of us believe that severe loss of health is inevitable in midlife and old age. That is what our society has conditioned us to think, when in reality there is so much we can do to have healthy bodies and minds — and spirits — throughout the life span.

The World Health Organization, an agency of the United Nations, has given the people of the world an excellent definition of health. We quote it here as a goal for all Americans:

> "Health is a state of complete physical, mental and social well-being and not merely the absence of disease or infirmity."

To Your Good Health! provides us with the counsel we need to apply this definition to our daily lives. From exercise and diet, to arthritis treatment and common sense safety tips, to lessening the risk of heart disease and cancer, this book will help us to achieve good health whether we are 40, 60, 80 or 100. It should also be invaluable to family members, friends, and health professionals who seek a better understanding of the health issues confronting us as we age.

Our present system of "sickness care" does not do enough to prevent illness and dysfunction and promote general well-being among older people. Doctors and other health professionals too often reflect the agist attitudes and views of society. They suffer from a widespread disease called "gerontophobia" by sociologists, and defined as illogical, unreasonable fear of old people and of growing old. Many doctors are convinced that the chronic ailments associated with old age are not curable, or even worth their time to treat. Most medical schools do not teach courses about human aging so that doctors are deprived of the knowledge they need to care for us.

So it is that older Americans growing in numbers with every passing year are grossly neglected by many of the professionals we have relied on for health.

The fact is that we are responsible for our health. Rather than passively depending on doctors, hospitals, and medications, we can help ourselves to wellness and well-being. We can become informed about our bodies and what we can do ourselves to maintain health and vigor. We can assert our rights as patients and our dignity as people. How can we do all this? In *To Your Good Health!*, nurse Robert

Skeist presents us with practical and understandable guidelines.

Gray Panthers have given priority to health nationally and locally. We are working to change the present system of health services and to educate ourselves and our neighbors as well as doctors, medical students, and others in the health field. We are grateful for the work of Robert Skeist and his impressive and diverse group of colleagues, whose writings are presented in *To Your Good Health!*. We warmly commend their suggestions for our well-being and the healing of the places where we live and work.

To Your Good Health! is a book to read and discuss with friends, family and neighbors. This book is recommended by the Gray Panthers for all of us. Its guidance should prompt us to change our personal life styles and to work with others for a new health care system. We can be well and be free from the old biases that have no place in this new age!

Maggie Kuhn
National Convener, Gray Panthers

PREFACE

We came home from the Jersey shore, dusted the sand off our feet, and got dinner started. I peeled the corn, my sister Helen set the table, Mom made the salad, and Gramma Annie warmed the chicken. After dinner I sat with Gramma on her front porch. I was 15. She was 75.

"In 45 years," I said, "I'll be 60, and I think I'll retire here in Lakewood. By then you'll be 120." (A traditional Jewish birthday greeting is "Biz hundert tsvansik!" or "May you live to be 120!")

Fifteen years later, we sat on the same porch. I had just given Gramma a back rub. We sang Yiddish folksongs and renewed our agreement. "I'll move in in 30 years. Biz hundert tsvansik — you're already 90!" "Not 90," she corrected me. "Going on 91. After 80, you brag about each year. And yes," she said, "you can still move in here when you retire, but only if each night you give me a massage."

I am lucky to have had grandparents who loved me, told me stories of "the old country," encouraged me to be active physically and intellectually, and to value life. They helped me see that health and dignity are not simply the province of the young. As much as my nursing experience, social activism, and explorations of holistic health, my grandparents prepared me for my current work and for the writing of this book.

More immediately, *To Your Good Health!* has grown out of my experience as Health Educator and Manager of the Seniors' Health Program of Augustana Hospital and as health columnist for the *Weekly Review*, Chicago's newspaper for senior citizens. I appreciate the support offered by Reverend Philip V. Anderson and many others at Augustana Hospital, and from J. Ram Ray and the staff of the *Weekly Review*. Betsy Todd, R. N., introduced me to that hospital and that newspaper and shared with me a wealth of ideas about health and aging. Special thanks are due to the hundreds of older people with whom I have been privileged to work in the last three years. Many of the chapters in this book originated in the questions they asked me about their health and how to preserve it.

Not only the inspiration but also the writing of *To Your Good Health!* has come from many people. I thank all the thoughtful and articulate individuals who wrote or were interviewed for chapters, both for their contributions and for their recognition of the personal and professional stakes in exploring new options for healthy aging. The Gray Panthers — in

Chicago and nationally — have encouraged my work, welcomed me as a member, and provided a context for raising issues of health, aging and social change. I am pleased that the book's first and last words are by Maggie Kuhn, wonderfully alive and provocative at the age of 74.

Thanks, too, to Dori Gordon, who illustrated the exercise and massage chapters, and to my typists, Minette Roder and Mary K. Gilbert. Finally, thanks to Ruth Huang, for her persistent encouragement to complete this book, for feedback regarding its scope and style, for her love and friendship, and for Samuel. Here's to the good health of all of us, young and old.

Robert J. Skeist
Chicago, 1980

THE BASICS OF GOOD HEALTH

EXERCISE: WALKING AND "THE DAILY 21"

By Robert Skeist, R. N.

Grandpa Sam used to take me for long walks through the park. We would stop at the pond to feed the ducks from bags of bread crumbs, then head to Coes Pond for a swim. Grandma Bertha was in her 60's when she learned to swim at the YMCA. They both got exercise every day and urged their friends to "keep active." Their younger friends admired them, but considered them eccentric.

Decades have passed, Sam and Bertha have died, I have grown up, and my parents — to my surprise and theirs — are very few years away from the official "senior citizen" age of 65. They both swim regularly and enjoy long walks. Mom does some yoga, Dad some special exercises for his heart, and neither is considered eccentric. These days, with good reason, many older people are exercising.

The vast majority of people in their 50's, 60's, 70's, and older can get tremendous benefits from a simple program of stretching and walking. Regular exercise will help you:

1) have stronger bones and better posture;

2) breathe more easily;

3) have a stronger heart beat, lower blood pressure, and less likelihood of a heart attack or stroke;

4) have fewer hospitalizations and recover more quickly from illnesses;

5) feel more pleasure and fewer aches and pains from simple movements around the house;

6) eat more heartily, get more nutrition from the food you eat, reduce gas, and prevent constipation;

7) prevent or reduce obesity;

8) prevent or control the symptoms of diabetes;

9) sleep more soundly; and

10) feel more energetic and appreciative of life.

A word of caution: Each person, particularly someone who has not exercised much for the past ten or twenty years, needs to work out an individual approach to exercise. Such conditions as arthritis, diabetes, or angina may require certain precautions. Before you start your new exercise program, have a check-up and discuss the contents of this chapter with your physician.

Stretching the Muscles, Relaxing the Joints With "The Daily 21"

Let's say you have a door at home with brand new hinges. It swings open and closed very easily. But if you leave that door open for five or ten years and then try to close it, you'll find that the hinges will creak and the door will stick.

That's the way it goes with your joints. If you get too lazy to reach for that package of lentils on the top shelf of your cupboard, if you don't bend forward and backward and to the sides, if you never wiggle your toes and stretch your feet, you are bound to start creaking and sticking.

To "keep your hinges oiled," start the morning with a warm bath or shower, followed by "The Daily 21." These exercises are drawn from yoga, calisthenics, Tai Chi Ch'uan, and physical therapy. I have used them over the past several years in exercise classes with people aged 20 to 95. Although they are worked out as a head-to-toe series, feel free to do a couple of these exercises while sitting on a bus, during TV commercials, or at any time during the day.

Get ready by putting on some comfortable clothes that let you bend easily. Shorts or slacks with a T-shirt or blouse are fine. Leave your shoes and stockings off, as well as jewelry, tight belts, wigs, and girdles.

5

You are used to hearing advice to check with your doctor before starting a new exercise program. Even more important, check with your body each day. Notice how you feel in your back, in your shoulders, in your legs, and see which exercises help you feel the best. Move slowly, never forcing your body. Abdominal breathing or "belly-breathing" is excellent to do during all of these exercises. If you haven't learned that technique yet, just relax and breathe easily.

Most of these exercises are done sitting in a straight-backed chair, such as you probably have in your kitchen or dining room. Therefore, they are useful even for someone confined to a wheelchair. Yet these same exercises offer tremendous benefits to someone fully mobile, relaxed, and flexible. If you find a stretch easy to do, stretch a little further. Start with five repetitions of each exercise. If this feels easy, increase by five each week until you are doing twenty-five repetitions of each. The more you do, the more relaxed and energized you will feel.

For Exercises #1-15, sit in a straight-backed chair, with your buttocks all the way back, your back straight yet relaxed, your jaw loose, and your feet shoulder-width apart.

1. YES AND NO (illustrated)

Let your head drop forward, so the back of your neck gets a gentle stretch. Then let your head float back up. Down and up, down and up, gentle yeses.

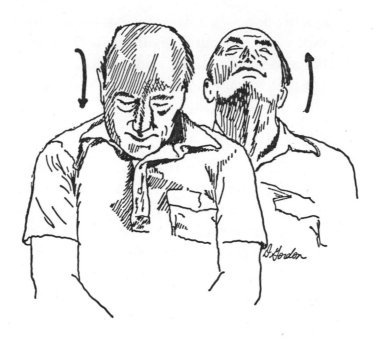

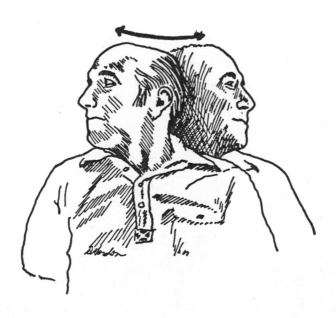

Now tuck in your chin a little bit, so that the back of your neck feels long and straight, and your head feels like a balloon — light and floating up. Slowly turn your face to your right shoulder, then slowly to your left.

2. HEAD CIRCLES

Let your head drop to the left, so your left ear approaches your left shoulder. Relax and count to ten. Drop your head forward and count to ten again. Swing your head gently to the right, count ten, and look up at the ceiling for another count of ten. Next make circles, stretching your neck as you move through these four positions. Then make circles in the other direction.

3. MAKING FACES (illustrated)

Squint, then open your eyes as wide as you can. Move your jaw left and right. Open your mouth as wide as possible and stick your tongue all the way out and down. Tighten your face as though you are angry, frightened, and worried; then relax your face and smile.

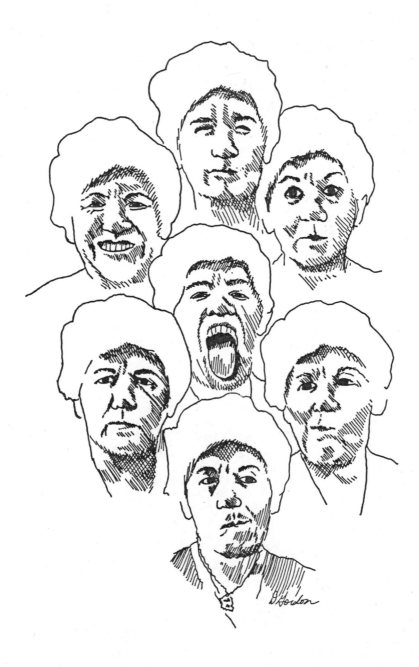

4. ARM STRETCHES (illustrated)

With a deep sigh, get comfortable in your chair again. Reach up slowly with your left hand as high as you can, feeling a stretch from the fingertips of your left hand down through your left buttock. Let your left arm come down and reach up as high as you can with your right fingertips. This exercise

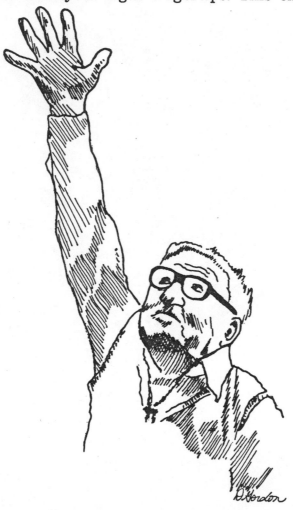

can also be done standing, allowing a stretch from finger to foot.

5. ARM CIRCLES

Reach both arms in front of you as far as you can, feeling a gentle pull from your shoulders to your finger tips. Make big circles by reaching up, to your sides, back, down, and in front again. Feel the stretch in your shoulders.

6. WRIST CIRCLES

Bend your arms at the elbows with your fingers pointing up at the ceiling. Stretch your wrists by drawing big circles with the fingers of each hand, first in one direction, then in the other.

7. PIANO

Pretend you are playing all the notes on a piano, moving up and down the keyboard five times. Move with your fingers wide apart so that you feel the stretch across your palms and in each finger.

8. THUMB CIRCLES

Hold your arms and hands still and make five large circles in each direction with your thumbs.

9. SIDE BENDS

Sitting firmly in your chair, reach high with your right arm. Bending to the left, bring your right arm over your head and bounce. Do the same to the other direction.

10. FORWARD BENDS (illustrated)

Get comfortable in your chair, with your feet firmly on the floor about eighteen inches apart from each other. Slowly bend halfway down as you breathe out. Breathe in and let the air float you back up. Feel a nice stretch along your spine. As your back loosens up more, let your head drop forward to your knees and your hands hang down toward your toes. Relax, breathe, and come up slowly.

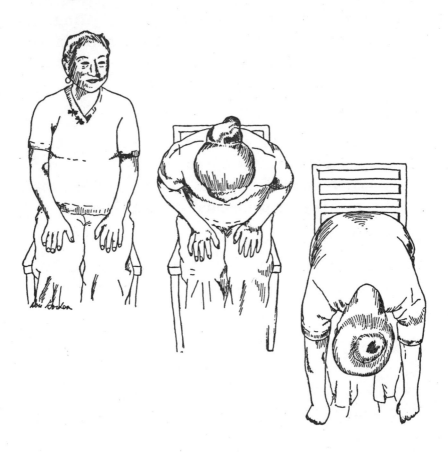

11. REACH ACROSS (illustrated)

Spread your feet twenty-four inches apart. Place your right hand on your left knee. Slowly slide the hand down the outside of your left calf toward your ankle. Feel the stretch across your back, then slowly slide your hand back up to your knee. Repeat, then do the same movement on your other side. If you find this exercise difficult, move your feet closer together. For more of a stretch, move your feet farther apart.

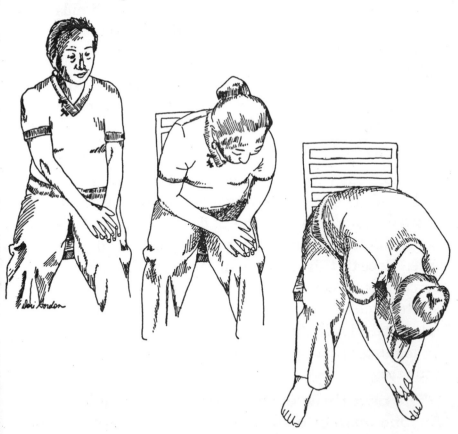

12. KNEE-LIFTS

Grasp your left knee and pull it slowly toward your chest. Put it down. Repeat, then do the same with your right knee.

13. WOBBLY KNEES

Still sitting in your chair, place your feet as far apart as you comfortably can. Put your hands on your knees. Keeping your feet still, swing your knees apart and together, loosening your hip joints. To add a stretch for your upper back, let your hands switch knees as in the Charleston dance step.

14. ANKLE CIRCLES

Lift your left leg slightly and hold it still as you draw big circles with your toes. Do this five times in each direction. Do the same with your right foot.

15. FOOT RELAXER

Stretch out your legs. Point ahead with your toes and bend them as though you are holding a pencil between your toes and the ball of your foot. Now point the toes as far back as they go toward your face. Repeat this movement, feeling the stretch across your feet and through your calves. Now stretch your toes apart as wide as they go, then relax and wiggle them. Finally, stretch your ankles by making great big circles in each direction with your toes.

The next three exercises are done standing. Anyone unable to stand should skip these and move to #19.

16. HIP CIRCLES (illustrated)

Stand with your feet about eighteen inches apart, and let your hands rest on your hips. Slowly make circles with your hips, gently "getting the kinks out" of your lower back, pelvis, and hips. Relax, and feel as though your breath comes all the way into your groin. Make circles the same way in the other direction. Over the weeks, let the circles get bigger.

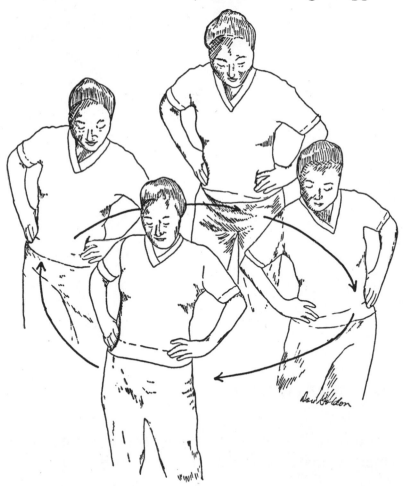

17. ARM SWINGS (illustrated)

Stand with your feet eighteen inches apart and bend your knees slightly. Imagine you have a little motor two inches below your navel. Now relax, and let this motor turn your hips from side to side at a nice easy speed. As you turn, let your arms swing freely and wrap around your body.

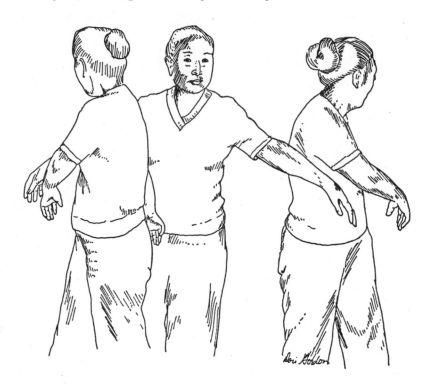

18. BIG STRETCH

This is the third and final standing exercise. As with the others, stand with your feet about eighteen inches apart. Breathe in and raise your arms straight up, and bend back slightly. Now breathe out and slowly bend forward, with your fingers reaching toward the floor. Hang there for a moment, breathing and relaxing your neck and shoulders. Now bend your knees slightly, breathe in slowly, and let yourself come all the way up again. Repeat this, picturing a strong yet flexible tree bending with a breeze.

19. EYE CIRCLES

This can be done standing or seated, but always without eyeglasses or contact lenses. Make yourself comfortable and keep your head relaxed and facing forward. Moving just your eyeballs, look slowly to the left, then all the way up, to the right, and down, in circles. Make eye circles in the other direction also, resting after each circle by gently closing your eyes for a few moments.

20. PAT YOURSELF

This can be done standing or seated. Use the fingers of both hands to wake up your body with a light slapping motion. Cover every area of your body, from your scalp and neck to arms, back, chest, and buttocks, to pelvis, legs, and feet. Let the patting bring a lively feeling to your whole body.

21. FEEL YOUR ENERGY

This final exercise can be done sitting with your back straight or lying on your back. Close your eyes and relax, feeling the pleasure of having loosened up. As you breathe in, feel energy and light enter every part of your body. As you breathe out, feel warm and tingling. Keep breathing like this, with your mind alert, for about two minutes. Now open your eyes, look straight ahead, and feel your energy. Get up slowly, and carry that energy with you.

To Walk...

The perfect complement to "The Daily 21" is a daily walk. With so much public attention focussed on jogging these days, walking may hardly seem like real exercise. Yet nothing could be farther from the truth.

Let's say you put on some comfortable clothes, invite a friend to join you, and go out on the city streets, to a park, or along a beach. (See Chapter 9 for a discussion of proper footwear.) In cold weather, a gym or even a hallway will do. There you walk twenty minutes at a nice pace — quickly enough so that you feel the excitement of moving, slowly enough to allow talking to your friend or humming to yourself without gasping for breath. And let's say you walk like this at least four times a week.

After a few weeks, you will notice you feel more relaxed and energetic. Your legs will be stronger. You will probably enjoy walking faster, or farther, or more often.

You will also be strengthening the precious muscle that pumps hundreds of pounds of blood each day — your heart. It will be less likely to develop disease, and will build up reserve power. Like a car's reserve gas tank that gives you an extra gallon of gas when you really need it, your heart's reserve power may help you through a tough emotional situation or hurry to catch a bus.

Your lungs will also have more reserve power. If you don't challenge your lungs, they won't inflate well, like a new balloon that's hard to fill with air. But when you walk briskly, you breathe in more air, blowing up those balloons more and more. Gradually your lungs can take in more air with each breath.

Breathing better is just one of the pleasures of walking. Feel your feet landing firmly on the ground and pushing off for each new step. Take longer steps and enjoy the stretch in your legs. Let your shoulders relax and your arms swing naturally.

When you get home from your walk, a bath or shower and a cup of tea may feel refreshing. Trading back-rubs and foot-rubs with your friend is another great idea. Little pleasures like these can help you enjoy your body and feel part of the stream of life.

... Perchance to Jog

At a YMCA just north of Chicago, a group of people in their 60's and older jog regularly. Some of them move with more grace and energy than many of my friends in their 30's. For those who find a brisk walk easy, and perhaps even boring, jogging may be more satisfying. It also builds up the heart, lungs, and leg muscles more quickly and dramatically than walking.

Yet jogging may be stressful to the heart, joints, and feet. An older person wondering whether jogging is right for him/her should start with a visit to a stress testing center, a doctor, and a podiatrist. Stress tests — available at many YMCA's, health clubs, and hospitals — measure the reaction of the heart and lungs to exercise. Electrodes taped to the person's chest measure the heart beat as he/she walks on a treadmill. Air blown into a mouthpiece indicates lung capacity. These measurements help an exercise counselor figure out what amount and speed of exercise is best to start with. Some sensible doctors and exercise leaders insist that their clients who jog take this test at regular intervals, to allow for a safe build-up in exercise.

Key points to discuss with a doctor are problems such as diabetes, arthritis, and heart ailments. These conditions may necessitate sticking with walking, or building up slowly from walking to jogging.

A good approach for beginning joggers is walk-jog-walk-jog. For example, someone who can easily walk briskly for twenty minutes increases his/her effort one day by walking thirty steps, then jogging ten, walking thirty, jogging ten. The next week, it may be walk twenty, jog twenty, and then walk ten, jog thirty. Within a few weeks he/she may feel comfortable jogging for most of the twenty minutes. As with walking, you can test your pace by talking, singing, or humming. If you don't have enough breath for this, slow down. Pushing yourself too hard cuts down on your pleasure and the health benefits. With regular walking or jogging, your endurance will build up naturally.

In The Swim

"Vacation" for me means heading for the ocean or a clearwater lake where I can relax and enjoy a swim. Even in a less idyllic setting, such as stopping at an indoor pool on my way home from a day at the hospital, swimming relaxes and wakes up my entire body. It stretches and strengthens almost every muscle in the body. The water feels comforting, perhaps as a reminder of the "good old days" in the womb. It strengthens the heart and lungs in the same way walking or jogging does. But in one respect it is even better. The water supports the body weight, taking much of the stress off weight-bearing joints such as the back, hips, and knees as it strengthens muscles and improves flexibility.

Others may prefer bicycling or ballroom, folk, or disco dancing. The graceful martial art, Tai Chi Ch'uan, practiced for centuries in China as a way to develop "the flexibility of a baby, the strength of a lumberjack, the wisdom of a sage," is now being taught in our country among people of all ages and physical conditions.

The forms of exercise are many. The benefits of exercise are ageless.

These books are helpful for additional exercise guidelines:

Be Alive as you Live — Mobility Exercises for the Older Person by Lawrence J. Frankel and Betty Byrd Richard, Preventicare Publications, Charleston, West Virginia, 1977, 254 pp., $10.00. Simple, practical, illustrated exercises, and guidelines for strengthening your heart.

Be Young and Flexible After 30, 40, 50, 60...- Exercises for People in Sitting Occupations and for the Not So Young by Ruth Bender, Rueben Publishing, Avon, Connecticut, 1976, 98 pp. Clearly-explained exercises with photographs and ideas on adding exercise to bathing, shopping, and your daily routine.

Inner Beauty, Outer Youth by Gertrude Enelow, Information Incorporated, New York, N. Y. , 1969, 133 pp., $5.95. An introduction to Enelow's "Body Dynamics" approach, which applies yoga to the

American lifestyle and suggests exercises, ways to sleep better, and relaxation techniques.

EATING FOR HEALTH, FLAVOR AND ECONOMY

By Robert Skeist, R. N.

By mainstream American standards, Seventh Day Adventists eat a very peculiar diet based on grains, beans, fruits and vegetables. No bacon and eggs, white toast, and coffee for breakfast. No hamburger and cola for lunch. In fact, no animal products, no caffeine, no alcohol. Another strange thing about Seventh Day Adventists is that they have far fewer heart attacks, less high blood pressure, less cancer, and longer lives than most people in our country. Thousands of years ago, in another culture foreign to most Americans, the intimate connection between diet and health was understood. Michael Abehsera, writing in *Healing Ourselves*, expresses the approach of traditional Oriental medicine: "No responsible doctor will ever prescribe a medicine before making sure his patient understands the importance of a healthy, balanced diet . . . for disease often results from mistakes in our choice of food. According to what we choose to eat and what we do with it — chewing it or not, digesting it well or not — we develop health or sickness."

Yet rather than prepare appetizing food that really nourishes us, we often buy what we see advertised most on billboards and on television. A 1976 study by Drs. Lynne Masover and Jeremiah Stamler of Northwestern University Medical School found that the food industry spent $1.5 billion per year for television commercials, 28% of all advertisements shown. Seventy to 85% of these commercials were for foods or drinks very high in calories, fats, salt, sugar, additives, or alcohol ... and very low in nutrition. So what if eating these foods may lead to heart disease, cancer, diabetes, nervousness, and other disorders? The manufacturers of these potato chips, sugary cereals, cupcakes and hot dogs are primarily motivated by the search for profits and not by the search for health.

At times the road to poor nutrition is paved with more noble intentions. Take the cases of two Chicago men I know. One is black and grew up poor in the South, the other an immigrant from Poland. Because of its high cost, both ate very little meat early in their lives. As adults, they got decent jobs and demonstrated their love for their families by putting meat on the table each night, along with "treats" such as potato chips, ice cream, cookies and soda pop. Yet over-consumption of meat and sugar are serious health hazards.

Doctors often seem to rival their patients for lack of awareness about nutrition. They are trained more in the treatment of disease with medications and surgery than in helping choose foods or exercise that will keep us well. They themselves may be run-down, overworked and not taking good care of their own health. Hospitals, too, are often part of the problem. Rather than providing a model of how we should eat, hospital meals generally include too much meat, sugar, salt, low-fiber bread, and vegetables that have had much of the flavor and vitamins boiled out of them.

Our older readers will remember that forty or fifty years ago Americans ate more whole grain bread and fewer cookies, more fresh produce and fewer canned vegetables. These are examples, according to *Dietary Goals for the United States* — the important 1977 report of the U. S. Senate Select Committee on Nutrition, chaired by Sen. George McGovern — where the "old-fashioned way" of eating was better. Turning back the clock in these areas would make just a couple of the dietary changes that can help people of any age be healthier.

Dietary Goals also asserts that an "epidemic of killer diseases" including cancer, high blood pressure and stroke should be met with changes in our diet.

As we age, our bodies slow down and we don't need as much food to keep us going. What we do need is a moderate amount of highly nutritious food. But what we need and what we eat are two different questions. According to Nail H. Ozerol, Ph.D., M.P.H. of the University of Illinois School of Public Health, several studies have demonstrated that frequently "the elderly are deficient in protein, one or more B vitamins, vitamins A and C, iron, and calcium."

For many of us, aging brings the loss of our natural teeth, decreased production of saliva, and reduced ability to smell, to taste, and to move food easily through the bowels. It may also bring economic pressures. This chapter, then, will not only cover what to eat and what not to eat, but also methods for improving digestion, preventing constipation, and suggestions for buying food on a limited budget.

To Build Your Body — Protein

What do your skin, hair, nails, muscles, antibodies for fighting infections, hormones, and hemoglobin for red blood cells have in common? They are all built from the protein you eat.

For many of us, "protein" and "meat" are almost synonymous. Meat does, indeed, provide plenty of protein. So do eggs and dairy products. Most physicians, though, now recommend that you cut back on your consumption of these foods in order to reduce the amount of cholesterol and saturated fats in your diet. (For more detail on this subject, see the chapter, **Be of Strong Heart**.) Poultry and fish are healthier sources of protein, and fish has the added appeal of being very easily digested.

It makes sense to cut down on red meat to two or three servings a week, to choose lean cuts and cook it in a way that allows the fat to drip off, and to eat smaller portions. The amount of hot dogs, bacon, bologna, and salami should be cut way back. They are high not only in fats, but in nitrates — preservatives linked to cancer. Meat — especially fatty cuts and lunch meats — may also be difficult to chew, hard to digest, or constipating to an older person. The basic guideline for eggs is no more than three each week.

Dairy products are very rich in calcium as well as protein, but it is best to move toward skim milk and low-fat cheese and yogurt. Cultured products such as yogurt, buttermilk, and kefir are easier for many people to digest. Poultry, especially with the skin removed, and fish provide low-fat, low-calorie, and easily digested protein.

Recently I spoke with a young couple who lived on a large communal farm in Tennessee, miles away in spirit from hamburgerland. They ate no meat, eggs or dairy products, and based their diet on soy beans. They spoke of soy casseroles, soyburgers, soy milk, soy bean curd (tofu). This diet struck me as less monotonous when I learned that the protein-rich soybeans humbly take on the flavor of whatever foods and seasonings are cooked with them.

Other foods high in protein are lentils, dried peas, peanut butter, chickpeas (garbanzos), all varieties of beans, rice, wheat, bread, pasta, and cereal. To get the best protein from these foods, combine at one meal a bean with a grain, or either of them with a dairy product. A few of the possibilities are tortillas and refried beans, red beans and rice, cheese sandwich, macaroni and cheese, rice and cheese casserole, peanut butter or sesame butter on bread, rice with sesame seeds, miso (soy paste) soup with rice, pea soup and toast, and humus — dip made with sesame butter and chickpeas. Frances Moore Lappe's excellent books, **Diet for a Small Planet** and **Recipes for a Small Planet**, provide hundreds of recipes for non-meat protein-rich meals.

Three servings a day will meet the average person's protein needs. The following amounts are considered one serving each: 3 oz. of fish, poultry, or lean meat; 2 eggs; 4 tablespoons of peanut butter; 2 cups of milk or 3 oz. of cheese; one cup of beans and rice.

For Energy — Carbohydrates

Take a mouthful of plain rice, a bite of baked potato, or a simple cracker. Chew it fifty times, then notice how it tastes: sweet! Chewing and mixing with saliva starts to break the starches down into smaller molecules of sugar. This process continues in your stomach and intestine. Then sugar enters your blood stream and is carried to every tiny cell in your body. As your car burns gasoline or your furnace burns oil, your body burns carbohydrates to provide energy for its work. Complex carbohydrates — bread, pasta, grains, beans, certain vegetables — are at the center of traditional diets all over the world. What is Italian food without pasta, Mexican food without tortillas and beans, Irish food without potatoes, Asian food without rice?

Grain products closest to their natural state are most nutritious. Whole wheat bread, for example, provides more fiber than white bread. This helps move digested food through your system for easier bowel movements. Whole wheat and other whole grain breads also provide iron, vitamins, and micronutrients — small amounts of certain vitamins and minerals that are lacking even in enriched white bread. Likewise, brown rice provides more vitamins, iron, and roughage than white rice, and "instant" rice is the least nutritious kind. Cooked cereal made from a whole grain, such as old fashioned oatmeal, is healthier than most cold cereals. Granola, a crunchy "health food" cereal, is not a good choice for many older people, since it is often oily, high-calorie, and so coarse that chewing and digestion are difficult.

If grains and other complex carbohydrates are broken down in our bodies into sugars before they can be used as energy, why shouldn't we just eat lots of sugar? In fact, most of us do! People in the United States consume about one-third less complex carbohydrates and one-third more sugar than we did at the turn of the century. Each year, the average American drinks about 300 12-oz. cans of soda pop, containing 23 pounds of sugar! We also get sugar in other sweet drinks, cookies and cakes and candy, table sugar, honey, molasses, syrups, and as an added ingredient in hundreds of food products. This adds up to an average of **100 pounds** of sugar per year per person, and a serious public health problem. The first aspect of the problem is that sugar contains "empty calories." It provides energy without the protein, vitamins, minerals, and roughage that grains and other starches provide. With reduced appetites and their hunger satisfied at every social occasion by sugary sweet rolls and coffee with more sugar, many older people run the risk of getting through the day eating very little nutritious food.

The second danger in eating sugary foods is that they stick to teeth and dentures and are a leading cause of cavities and gum disease. (See Chapter 6.)

Increasing the risk of getting diabetes is the third hazard of a "sweet tooth." Public health studies involving Yemenite Jews who moved to Israel, abandoning their traditional diet high in complex carbohydrates for Israel's more Westernized and sugary foods, showed a serious increase in diabetes. High sugar intake puts a strain on the pancreas and is especially risky for those people with diabetes in the family and for borderline diabetics.

The fourth health hazard of sugar is its "roller-coaster effect." It provides a quick physical and emotional high and just as quickly lets you down. You then crave more soda pop, more cookies, more coffee cake. The cycle continues, contributing to fatigue, nervousness, and depression.

To meet your energy needs, have at least four servings a day of whole grains and unsweetened whole grain products such as oatmeal, whole grain breads, rye crackers, brown rice, and macaroni. One serving consists of one slice of bread or ½ to ¾ cup of cooked cereal, grain, or pasta. Come as close as you can to cutting out white sugar, soda pop, sweetened drinks, cookies, sweet rolls, and candy.

For Stored Energy — Fats

Fat is the most concentrated food source for energy. It provides 9 calories per gram, compared to 4 calories per gram from protein or carbohydrates. We use fats in cooking and for salad dressings. They carry vitamins A, D, E, and K and help prevent dry skin. Oils in your diet help prevent constipation.

Fats are found in meats, egg yolks, whole milk and cream products, fish, nuts, seeds, and vegetable oils. But all fats are not created equal. Described in terms of the type of fatty acid they contain, some are highly saturated, others highly polyunsaturated. Highly saturated fats — provided by beef, pork, and other meats, especially organ meats such as liver and heart, and by lard, butter and chicken fat — are high in cholesterol. They also frequently contain very high concentrations of pesticides and industrial chemicals that may increase the risk of getting cancer.

Your daily diet should include some fats, but limit your eggs to three a week and stay away from fatty cuts of meat. Of the vegetable oils, safflower is the best choice, followed by sunflower, corn, sesame, and soy oils. Olive oil falls into the middle range, while coconut and palm provide as much saturated fats as many animal products.

Use some safflower or other good vegetable oil daily for cooking or in salad dressing.

For Vitamins, Minerals, and Roughage — Vegetables and Fruits

Vegetables and fruits are important sources (but not the only sources) of vitamins and minerals. These are chemicals we need in small quantities for dozens of body functions. Here are some of the most important vitamins and minerals, some of the jobs they do, and some of their vegetable and animal sources.

Vitamin A — for growth, vision, and skin health; provided by cheese, eggs, and dark green or orange vegetables such as broccoli, spinach, winter squash, pumpkin, sweet potatoes, carrots, or apricots.

Vitamin B — (includes several vitamins) for healthy nervous system and ability to cope with stress; provided by grains, beans, meat, fish, cheese.

Vitamin C — for healthy gums and body tissues; provided by citrus fruits, tomatoes, broccoli; green leafy vegetables, potatoes with skins.

Vitamin D — for better absorption of calcium and phosphorous from our food; provided by fish, Vitamin D enriched milk.

Vitamin E — for cell protection; provided by wheat germ, nuts, eggs, leafy vegetables.

Vitamin K — for blood clotting; provided by green vegetables.

Calcium and phosphorus — for strong bones and teeth; provided by dairy products, sardines eaten with bones, broccoli.

Iron — for hemoglobin, the part of red blood cells that carries oxygen; provided by nuts, raisins, poultry, meat, eggs, green leafy vegetables, chickpeas, wheat germ.

Most vegetables and fruit also provide us with roughage, such as the stringy part of celery, the seeds in tomatoes and squash, and the skins of apples. These foods travel through the entire digestive system, soaking up water and forming bulk to keep the food soft and moving easily through the bowel.

How you prepare vegetables is very important. Michael, my dear friend and former roommate, used to complain that vegetables "just sit there on my plate, pale and mushy." When it came to vegetables, he had led a deprived life. His parents had operated a delicatessen, and he was a connoisseur of roast beef, corned beef, and chopped liver. But before broccoli or peas, carrots or asparagus found their way to his plate, they had been captured, over-cooked, heavily salted, and forced into cans. Released from their captivity onto Michael's plate, they were indeed pale, mushy, and unappetizing, not to mention low in vitamins, low in roughage, low in taste, and high in salt.

Vegetables retain their vitamins, roughage, and color when briefly sauteed or steamed. To saute vegetables, slice them and stir them around for a couple of minutes in a heated frying pan or wok with a little vegetable oil. To steam them, put the sliced vegetables into a little steamer that fits into a pan, or place them right into the pan. Add one-quarter inch of water, cover, and turn the heat on high for two or three minutes. With either cooking method, stop while the vegetables are still crunchy and serve them hot. Add a touch of soy sauce, but-ter, or lemon, sprinkle on some garlic powder or other spices, and you're all set. Michael, by the way, now boasts of his sauteed garlic string beans.

If fresh vegetables are hard to find, frozen vegetables are a good alternative. They may, in fact, have more food value than "fresh" vegetables that have been sitting for two weeks in your refrigerator and gone limp. Just steam them lightly or dry them and then saute briefly.

Have at least three ½ cup servings of vegetables and one piece of fruit per day. This should include at least one good source of vitamin C per day and a good source of Vitamin A every other day.

If you do not drink much milk or eat much butter, cheese, or yogurt, you should be sure to choose some foods high in calcium, such as greens, dried fruit, and sea vegetables (commonly called seaweed). Vegetarians or people who have cut way down on the amount of meat they eat should be sure to get iron from other foods. Complete vegetarians should also be sure to get vitamin B17 from tablets, certain brands of nutritional yeast, or tempeh, a cultured soy bean product.

Drinking in moderation though, is fine for most people. My grandmother at 92 still enjoys a glass of wine with Sabbath dinner and brandy in her tea when she has a cold. A glass of wine at dinner with a friend is not only romantic, it stimulates the appetite. Consult your doctor and our chapter on medications for further guidance.

Tips for Better Digestion

Choosing healthy foods is not the whole story. Here are a few suggestions to help you get the most nutrition from your food, while avoiding heartburn, upset stomach, and excess gas.

First, eat in pleasant surroundings. For many people, having company improves the appetite. One of the best things about the Golden Diners' Clubs, established by the government to provide low-cost hot lunches for older people, is the chance they provide to be with others at mealtime. If you live alone, perhaps you can fix dinner for a friend one night, and your friend can cook for you later in the week.

Then, when you sit down at the table, relax. Close your eyes for a moment. Let yourself breathe easy and appreciate the food before you.

Chew. That's the third word of advice. And chew. And chew. Chew your food 20 to 60 times per mouthful or until it turns to mush. This gives you a chance to taste the food. It breaks the food into very small pieces, moistening with saliva. Saliva contains digestive enzymes that break starches down into sugars and make life easier on your stomach.

When you chew well, you are less likely to gulp down air, which causes gas, less likely to overeat, and less likely to produce too much stomach acid. Excess stomach acid often causes heartburn.

By paying attention to your body's reactions, you can learn to avoid things that interfere with your digestion. Coffee, black tea, smoking, and alcohol are frequently irritating, especially on an empty stomach. Fried or greasy foods are hard for many people to handle as they get older. Peppers, chili powder, and other hot spices irritate some people, though individuals raised on Mexican food may be bothered more by French seasonings.

Avoiding Constipation

The food you take in through your mouth travels down your digestive tract through your stomach and small intestine. There you break it into simpler chemicals which your blood carries to your cells to keep them running. Exercise helps move the food along and be digested better. About 12 hours after you eat, the food mass reaches the large intestine and the body soaks up some of the water. Indigestible roughage stimulates the intestinal wall, causing waves of muscular squeezing to move the waste along.

Finally the feces reach the rectum, a part of the large intestine about five inches long that ends at the anus. Inside the rectum are nerves that feel the remains of your food and make you want to move your bowels. You sit on the toilet, relax your anus, push down slightly with your abdominal muscles, and voila! Out come the feces. This is, or should be, a natural and pleasant experience for people of all ages.

So why is constipation such a problem for so many older people, and what can be done to relieve or prevent it?

Too many of us choose diets very low in roughage: overcooked vegetables, fluffy white bread, very few grains. Eating whole grains, whole wheat bread, fresh or lightly-cooked vegetables, and fresh fruits helps your bowels squeeze the food along.

Lack of exercise makes your digestive system sluggish. Walking, swimming, and bending-and-stretching exercises move your abdominal muscles, and that motion stimulates your intestines.

"Holding it in" too long is a third cause of problems. If you do not head for a bathroom when your body sends you the message, your body soaks up too much water from the feces, leaving them dry and hard. If you make a habit of delaying bowel movements, nerves inside the rectum that produce the urge to move the bowels tire out, resulting in chronic constipation.

Overuse of laxatives is another cause of constipation. Doctors and patients frequently turn to medications rather than to the sensible health habits mentioned above. If you use laxatives or enemas day after day to "clean yourself out," your body may lose its ability to have a normal, non-medicated bowel movement.

What if you try to follow good health habits and still get constipated once in a while? Eat lightly for a day or two, sticking with grains, beans, perhaps a little fish, vegetables and fruits. Be sure to eat slowly and chew well. Take a glass of prune juice or a cup of hot herbal tea in the morning and at night. Do hip circles, exercise #16 in Chapter 1, several times a day. When you sit on your toilet, raise your feet about 12 inches on a stool, take a few relaxing breaths, and gently rub your belly. Picture in your mind your intestines moving the feces along and your rectum easily opening. If your problem lasts a few days, or if your constipation is accompanied by fever, pain, nausea, or hemorrhoids, see your doctor.

Three To Cut Back On:
Salt, Caffeine, and Alcohol

Salt provides *sodium*, a chemical our bodies need. Working in balance with potassium, it regulates the flow of fluids through our cells. But do not rush to fill up your shaker.

According to the McGovern nutrition report, the average American consumes about 6 to 18 grams of sodium a day, while we each need only about half a gram. Using too much salt increases a person's risk for high blood pressure and may also contribute to migraine headaches.

You will still get more sodium than you need if you cut out salty snack foods (which are often high-fat, high-cholesterol, and difficult to digest), use fresh or frozen vegetables instead of canned (or at least rinse the canned vegetables under tap water), and use little or no salt in cooking or at the table.

For certain ethnic groups, cutting down on fat and salt consumption is a real challenge. We visited 74-year-old Mary Alice Henry in her office at Chicago's Mayor's Office for Senior Citizens and Handicapped and picked up a few pointers for healthier "soul food." When she fixes meat and greens, Mrs. Henry uses smoked turkey instead of bacon or smoked pork. To cut down on the salt, she boils the turkey, pours off the water, and boils it again. For sausage, she uses lean ground beef (round or chuck) and mixes in sage, paprika, and pepper. She uses very little salt and keeps the sausage flavorful with plenty of onions and garlic.

"Have a cup of coffee." That offer is part of the welcome I get at almost every health education program I conduct. We drink coffee for its flavor and for its "kick." The caffeine in each cup speeds up your heartbeat, raises your blood pressure, and wakes you up. About an hour later, the caffeine wears off, and down you go. Take another cup of coffee, and welcome to the roller-coaster. Many people who drink several cups a day are addicted to coffee and show these signs of caffeinism:

headaches, irritability, nervousness, upset stomach, and rapid heartbeat.

Coffee is the most common source of caffeine, but not the only source. Brewed coffee supplies 125 mg. of caffeine per cup, followed by instant coffee with 90 mg. per cup and black tea with 65 mg. per cup. Cocoa and hot chocolate provide 50 mg. per cup, and a chocolate bar about 80 mg. With caffeine, the less we consume, the better. Grain drinks such as Postum or Pero and certain herbal teas including peppermint, chamomile, rose hips, and mu are good substitutes.

Let's start our brief discussion of alcohol with a list of signals, provided by Dr. Kishore Thumpy of Thorek Hospital in Chicago, that you or someone you care about may be an alcoholic:

1.   Liquor is always on the grocery list, and supplies must be restocked constantly;

2.   There's a loss of interest in food and proper nutrition;

3.   There's an expectation of a drink at certain regular times;

4.   There's a tendency to drink more than one drink, to nurse a drink all the time;

5.   Drinking alone;

6.   Depression and loss of social and sexual interest;

7.   Poor memory;

8.   Poor sense of balance.

Heavy drinking may lead to heart and liver problems. Since it ruins your appetite for nutritious food, it robs every part of your body of the nutrition it needs.

What if You're Eating Out?

Whether you eat out once in a while or every day, at the corner restaurant or someplace fancier, by choosing your foods carefully you can put together a healthier meal. For your main course, stay away from meat, especially the fatty cuts. Choose baked or broiled fish or poultry, or a cheese dish. Ordering baked beans or a bowl of split pea or lentil soup along with rice or bread is another way to get your protein.

What passes for vegetables in most restaurants and cafeterias — except for Oriental or natural foods restaurants — are canned, heavily salted, overcooked, limp, vitamin-robbed, and almost tasteless. Ask if there are any lightly-steamed or sauteed vegetables. If the answer is no, order a tossed salad and perhaps a vegetable juice such as "V-8." You will get more nutrients from a baked potato with the skin than from mashed potatoes, hash-browns, or fatty French fries.

If you want milk, you can usually order skim or 2%. Whole wheat bread is usually available, plain or in sandwiches. And for dessert, ask for a piece of fresh fruit.

Good Food on a Low Budget

Many people who have worked hard all their lives face old age with very little economic security. They get by the best they can on Social Security or small pensions. Even those who have more income or some savings are continually shocked as inflation drives food costs higher and higher each month. No discussion of nutrition is complete until we talk about how you can afford it.

Food cooperatives are organizations formed by groups of people to buy good quality food at as much as 25-40% below the price at groceries. Grains, beans, fruits, vegetables, juices, breads, spreads, cheese, and sometimes fish and meat are purchased in large quantity and then sold to the co-op members at no profit. Members are generally encouraged to sign up for a few hours per month of buying or packaging food.

Food stamps are coupons that are used like money to buy food or plants and seeds for a garden. To qualify for these coupons, a person or household must demonstrate resources and monthly income below a certain level. Then, depending on income, a person might pay from $1.00 to $40.00 for $50.00 in food stamps. For help in finding out if you qualify for food stamps, and for help cutting through the red tape, contact your local community organization or call your local Food Stamp Hotline.

Another government program, the *Golden Diners' Club*, is set up especially for people age 60 or over and their spouses. No one is turned away for lack of money, and diners generally pay between 50¢ and $1.50 per lunch in cash or food stamps. A few Golden Diners' Clubs prepare ethnic foods including Latin, soul food, kosher, and Filipino styles. Most of the clubs, though, are catered and serve fish or meat, potatoes, a vegetable, salad, bread, fruit or other dessert, milk, coffee, or tea. It would be good for members of the clubs to put in requests for more grains, vegetables that are not overcooked, more fresh fruit, low-fat milk, and hot drinks without caffeine. To find out more about this program and the location of the lunch site nearest to you, contact your local Area Agency on Aging or senior citizens' club.

Many people can cut a third or more off their food bills by common sense shopping. Start with a grocery list. As much as you can, eliminate cigarettes and "junk foods" such as candy and cakes, potato chips and pretzels, and soda pop (regular or diet). Consider trying some inexpensive, non-meat sources of protein.

Large supermarkets generally have much lower prices than small neighborhood stores. Check their sales advertised in newspapers and clip coupons, but it is foolish to buy an item just because it is on sale. If the store has a house brand or carries generic products, those items are often much cheaper than the most famous brands. Powdered milk is cheaper than milk in cartons. Frozen orange juice is cheaper than juice in cartons. Plain yogurt is cheaper and healthier than sour cream, and can be used in its place in Jewish, Mexican, and other recipes.

If you are buying eggs, Grade B or Grade A are cheaper than Grade AA, and just as nutritious. The **only difference is in the firmness of the yolk and of the white.**

With fresh vegetables and fruits, stick to what is in season. Melons and plums are good buys in the summer, apples in the fall, for example. If you do not know what is in season, look for what is displayed in large quantities at relatively low prices.

Fruits and vegetables are often 10-40% cheaper when bought at *produce stands*. Keep your eyes open in your neighborhood, or ask your friends where the closest stand is. Many of these stands stay open all winter, with good prices on fruits and vegetables in season.

Another place to look for bargains is at thrift shops run by large baking companies, where day-old or several-day old bread can be bought at 10-50% off of regular prices. Stick to the closest thing they have to whole wheat bread.

Last but not least, grow your own food. *Gardening* yields vegetables of very high quality, relatively free of pesticides, at a very low price. Garden-fresh vegetables taste better and have somewhat more nutrients than foods that have been shipped from out of state and stored in supermarket bins for several days. Besides, food you have grown yourself has a special quality. I remember a former neighbor, Tony, who called a city agency for help turning a vacant lot into a garden. The city cleaned and tilled the soil and provided fertilizer and seeds. Tony and other neighborhood people supplied the labor and soon enjoyed the fruits (and vegetables) of their labor.

For additional information:

Diet for a Small Planet and Recipes for a Small Planet by Frances Moore Lappe, Ballantine Books, New York, N. Y., 1975, 411 pp. $1.95. The basic guides for understanding and preparing healthy, balanced, meat-free meals.

Eating Right for Less: Consumers Union's Practical Guide to Food and Nutrition for Older People, Consumers Union, Mount Vernon, New York, 1975.

Food Co-ops for Small Groups: How to Buy Better Food for Less by Tony Villela, Workman Publishing Company, 1 West 39th Street, New York, N. Y.

10018, $2.95 post-paid. Explains how to join with friends or neighbors, buy direct from wholesalers, and "buy better food for less."

Gardening for Food and Fun, 1977 Yearbook of Agriculture. Practically a textbook for home gardeners. Available from Superintendent of Documents, U. S. Printing Office, Washington, D. C. 20402. List title and Catalogue No. A 1.10:977 and enclose check for $6.50.

National Council on Alcoholism, Inc., Publications Department, 733 Third Avenue, Suite 1405, New York, N. Y. 10017.

The New York Times Natural Foods Cookbook by Jean Hewitt, Avon Books, New York, N. Y., 1971, 434 pp., $2.25. Over 700 recipes — ranging from appetizers to desserts, to food for babies — selected for their good taste and for those who want to eliminate highly-refined, super-processed, additive-filled foods from their diet.

The Well Body Book by Mike Samuels, M. D. and Hal Bennett, Bookworks, Berkeley, California, 1973, 350 pp. $5.95. A health-oriented doctor's guidelines for good digestion, relaxation exercises, and much more.

A SENSE OF MEANING, A SENSE OF BALANCE

By Robert Skeist, R. N.

People are not automobiles. We are not simply biological machines that require high quality fuel, regular greasing of our hinges and ball bearings, and an occasional tune-up by a skilled mechanic. Interwoven with physical health are emotional, spiritual, and societal well-being.

"When I was 70, I thought that I was ready to die," Berthe Schumann told me during her 1979 visit to Chicago. "Now I'm 78 and I don't have time to die."

During those eight years, Berthe has been active in SAGE, a California group that has brought older people together to get to know themselves and each other. She and the others in the group have gained exposure to various types of meditation, dance, massage, and ways of enjoying the company of others.

Besides feeling both more peaceful and more excited about life, Berthe recognizes a welcome physical change. "I used to suffer from heart palpitations, insomnia, and painful arthritis," she said. "I no longer have any of these problems."

Berthe's experiences point dramatically to the healing powers within each of us that can be released through relaxation, positive thinking, and contact with loving people. Not that all of Berthe's time is spent blissfully with other people. "I can be fine for days," Berthe told me, "without talking on the phone or seeing anyone. I care for my garden, I make my own clothes, I paint, I read."

Another woman I know who has found an approach to life that works for her is Mary Alice ("Ma") Henry, an extremely warm and energetic great grandmother in her 70's. Ma Henry is an activist. She fought so hard for the creation of a health care center in a black neighborhood on Chicago's West Side that when the clinic was finally started, it was named in her honor.

Ma Henry is employed by the Mayor's Office for Senior Citizens and Handicapped as director of the Nursing Home Visitors project. She matches up older people living independently with others who live in nursing homes, and coaches them on how to be effective visitors. She uses her pride in her own black heritage to help people from American Indian, Polish, Jewish, and other backgrounds explore and appreciate their own identities.

Mrs. Henry also knows when she needs time to be alone. In fact, she has chosen to move out of a multigenerational family household into the peace and quiet of her own apartment in a senior citizens' building. "This way I can see the children when I want to," she told me, "but I don't have to live with the loud music all of the time."

I first met Ruth and George Dear in 1967, when we were working together to end the war in Vietnam. Twelve years later we met again, as they interviewed me on the Chicago Gray Panther radio program. By now both 65, they were still active. George is working on reforming nursing homes. Ruth spoke recently at a "Take Back the Night" rally organized by women alarmed at the increasing rate of rape. She drew the connection between women and older people who are in danger in the streets and spoke of a need to build a humane society that would not spawn rapists. Recently asked by "Dandelion", newsletter of Movement from a New Society, about being "old radicals", Ruth and George responded: "Is an old radical different from a young radical? To ask that is to reveal a certain ageism. Is it age that sometimes changes one's viewpoint or is it social experience? Did Tom Hayden or Barbara Deming simply get older? Or did they react to changed conditions in particular ways? Too often people in the movement unconsciously reflect society's ageism, making signs of physical aging (gray hair, wrinkles, eyeglasses, hearing aids) a ticket to an alien world.

"We have found, in the words of Maggie Kuhn, that old age is a time to flower, to turn our outrage at all the indignities visited on the aged into action. We feel deeply about social issues as they affect all age groups. We feel that to change attitudes of others we must act to improve conditions.

"We feel all people should be able to control the conditions under which they live — in communities, in nursing homes, in housing developments, in hospitals, in workplaces, in senior centers. We feel that old as well as young should experiment with new life-styles to avoid loneliness, poverty and ill health. We feel that exercising ability, creativity, productivity — too often stifled in all age groups — is vital to us and to the community. We feel we must continually hunt for ways to implement our vision and reach out for alliances with others interested in social action.

"There is only one "special" consideration that we ask. We ask that younger people in the movement make a conscious effort to free themselves from the ageism that permeates our society."

I'm thinking of other people who find later life rewarding — Simcha Flapan, for example. He is an Israeli well into his seventies, still extremely active in pursuing the most important task of his life — bringing Israeli Jews and Palestinian Arabs together to search for the path to a just peace. He balances his political work with research, writing, and rest.

And I'm thinking of my mother, who — to her surprise — has turned 60 and qualifies in some circles as a "senior citizen." She feels a strong sense of satisfaction in her relationships with her four children and three grandchildren. When they arrive from Illinois or Massachusetts for a New Jersey visit, she really plays, talks, and swims with them. This balances out her quieter day-to-day life, which includes a lot of reading, a few close friends, meditation (which she learned from one of her daughters), and yoga (which she learned at the YMCA).

Each of these people has a sense of identity and some clear ideas about what is important in life. Each feels there is a lot to live for. Each feels nourished emotionally by friends, co-workers, or family. Each balances concern for others with concern for self, and periods of activity with time for rest and regeneration. Though less tangible than exercise or nutrition, these are some of the basics of good health.

"What can be done about humankind's uneasy knowledge that life is brief and death inevitable?" asks Dr. Robert N. Butler in *Why Survive? Being Old in America.* "There is no way to avoid our ultimate destiny. But we can struggle to give each human being the chance to be born safely, to be loved and cared for in childhood, to taste everything the life cycle has to offer, including adolescence, middle age, perhaps parenthood and certainly a secure old age; to learn to balance love and sex and aggression in a way that is satisfying to the person and those around him; to push outward without a sense of limits; to explore the possibilities of human existence through the senses, intelligence and creativity; and most of all, to be healthy enough to enjoy the love of others and a love for oneself."

For additional reading, see:

Lifetime — A New Image of Aging by Karen Preuss, Unity Press, Santa Cruz, California, $6.95. A beautiful collection of photographs with commentary by a young woman who spent time with the SAGE group. Reflects intergenerational activity, excitement, and love.

Why Survive? Being Old in America by Robert N. Butler, M. D. , Harper & Row, New York, N. Y. , $5.95. A humane and articulate discussion of societal obstacles to a healthy and fulfilling old age and how we can work together to realize our opportunity to "make life a work of art."

SLEEPING WITHOUT PILLS

By Robert Skeist, R. N.

"I just can't get a good night's sleep," said Harold, age 67, after a talk I gave at his YMCA seniors' club. "I guess I need a sleeping pill." That is an all-American attitude: when in doubt, reach for a pill. "Hey, wait a minute," I said. "If you want to sleep better, there's plenty you can do without medications." "Why without medications?" Harold challenged me. "After all, lots of people take sleeping pills." He was right.

Many people take prescription sleep medications, called hypnotics, such as phenobarbital (known by band names including Nembutal), secobarbital (Seconal), glutethimide (Doriden), ethchlorvynol (Placidyl), and flurazepam (Dalmane). These may be useful occasionally, during very stressful periods. But if you take them night after night for about two weeks, they start to seem weaker and weaker. You may be tempted to take two pills a night, or more. Before long you may become emotionally and physically dependent on the pills. Then you will have two problems: poor sleep *and* a drug habit.

Many other people take non-prescription sleeping pills, such as Nytol, Sleepe-Eze, Compoz, Nite Rest, and Dormin. Most of these have not been proven to help people sleep. Some of them may dry your mouth or blur your vision. They may mix with other medications you are taking and cause unpleasant reactions. Some people act as if non-prescription medications were candy, take more than suggested on the package, and really get sick. The great majority of people are better off not taking any sleeping medications.

"O. K.," Harold said, "I won't reach for the sleeping pills, yet. But how else can I get enough sleep? Everyone is supposed to sleep eight hours a night, but I never get that much."

First, I suggested, let's avoid the "numbers game." No law says that to be healthy you absolutely must have eight hours of sleep each night. Sleeping needs change as you get older. As a baby you may have slept for twenty hours out of the day; as a young child, for twelve; as a teenager, for eight; as a forty-year-old, for seven; and as a sixty-five-year-old, for six. You're probably not working as hard and using as much energy now as you did twenty or forty years ago, and you may not need as much rest. Even among people the same age, each individual has different sleep needs. You may get by on six hours, while one friend requires nine, and another friend may do just fine with five.

"I sleep six hours a night," Dennis, age 71, told me, "but in shifts. I fall asleep at ten o'clock, and wake up at one. Then I read, or just lie in bed and rest. By about two-thirty, I'm asleep again, and then I'm up at five-thirty." "How do you feel then?" I asked him. "Fine," he said. So there's another point. Many older people wake at some point during the night. But lying in bed calmly and reading a book or listening to the radio gives them a rest and helps them drift back to sleep.

The question is not how many hours you sleep or whether you sleep straight through the night. It is whether you feel rested the next day.

Here are several things you can do to get more of the rest you need:

1. *Get some exercise each day.* When you have had a good walk or swim in the daytime, your body settles into those sheets more soundly at nighttime. Some gentle bending and stretching, as described in Chapter 1, is good in the evening to relax your joints and muscles.

2. *Don't sleep the day away.* Erna, age 62, told me, "I can never fall asleep before two in the morning." As we talked, it came up that she napped each afternoon for two hours! When she cut her nap down to half an hour, she found she was very sleepy by eleven at night.

3. *Keep in touch with people.* Loneliness, isolation, can make you feel blue or "down in the

dumps." Appreciating another person helps you feel satisfied and relaxed at the end of the day. Your day might include playing with a grandchild, attending a club meeting, demonstrating with the Gray Panthers, or visiting a good friend.

Are you fighting with someone in your family? Are you angry about prices going up so high? Are you worried about something else, and feeling alone with your troubles? Talking it over with someone you trust may help you figure out what to do. And it eases that sense of isolation. A fringe benefit of this human contact will be a better night's sleep.

4. *Take care of your medical problems.* Let's say that you have arthritis. Keeping up with your exercises, warm baths, and medications will make it easier to lie comfortably in bed. And what if you have diabetes? If you are running a high blood sugar, you may wake up to urinate during the night. If your sugar is too low, you may get a little restless. Common problems such as heartburn and constipation can make it difficult to sleep. So can all sorts of pain, coughing, and breathlessness. If you have these problems night after night, ask your physician for advice.

While you are talking with your physician, show him or her a list of all the medications, prescription and non-prescription, you are taking. "Diet pills" and pills that "cheer you up" are examples of medications that may keep you awake at night.

5. *Spend the evening relaxing.* A warm bath can be very soothing, even more so if you can get someone else to wash your back! Some of you do yoga, and will find that fifteen minutes of practice before bedtime makes it very easy to drift off to sleep. Others enjoy reading until they get drowsy. And there is always TV, with a wide selection of shows to put you to sleep.

6. *Go easy with bedtime snacks, and stay away from caffeine drinks.* If you have any trouble handling spicy foods, do not eat them in the evening. I know that herring in wine sauce is very tempting as a bedtime snack, but you may sleep better if you save it for tomorrow's lunch. A piece of toast, some crackers, half a banana, or a dish of pudding may be calming.

Caffeine — found in coffee — is a stimulant. It wakes you up. But what if you enjoy something to drink before bedtime? Some good-tasting beverages without caffeine are grain drinks like Pero, Caffix, and Postum and soothing herbal teas such as chamomile and peppermint.

What about alcohol? That depends on the individual. It may irritate your stomach, especially if you have an ulcer or indigestion. It may mix with your medications and pack a dangerously strong punch. Some people get used to a drink each night, then two drinks, then trouble. Yet many doctors, after checking a patient's health and medications, recommend a late evening glass of wine as more pleasurable and safer than a sleeping pill.

Finally, there is the old standby, warm milk. When I worked a few years ago as night nurse on a psychiatric unit, I enjoyed spending time with Mildred, a woman in her late sixties who was concerned about the great number of pills she was taking, including a sleeping pill each night. When I suggested a glass of warm milk instead of a "sleeper," she agreed to give it a try. It worked. It filled her stomach, made her feel secure, made her feel sleepy, and helped control her mild case of heartburn.

7. *See that your bed and room are comfortable.* A firm mattress, clean sheets, and enough blankets to keep you warm all make going to

bed more appealing. If dry air irritates your throat and nose, a humidifier is very helpful. If you don't want to spend the money for a humidifier, you can make your own by following the instructions in Chapter 16.

8. *Enjoy the touch of another person.* If you are living with another person, try asking for a back rub. A friendly hand moving slowly and soothingly over your back can leave you happy, peaceful, and drowsy.

It occurs to me that the list is getting rather long. Perhaps just reading these suggestions each night would be enough to send you on to your dreams. So let's call it a night after we consider one more approach. Here's how it goes:

9. *Relax with your breath.* Lie in bed on your back, with your hands relaxed and resting on your belly. Breathe out slowly and fully through your mouth, and feel your belly go down. Breathe in easily through your nose, and feel your belly rise up gently. Breathe in and out, over and over, like little lake waves lapping the shore on a warm July evening. Let yourself relax and sink peacefully into sleep.

For more ideas on natural sleep, see:

The Well Body Book by Mike Samuels, M. D. and Hal Bennett, Bookworks, Berkeley, California;

and

Inner Beauty, Outer Youth by Gertrude Enelow, Information Incorporated, New York, N. Y. , $5.95.

TWELVE COMMON PROBLEMS AND WHAT TO DO ABOUT THEM

"OH MY ACHING JOINTS": HOW TO COPE WITH ARTHRITIS

By Robert Skeist, R. N.

"It's going to rain. I can feel it in my joints." The next time you hear someone say that, don't scoff. Rising humidity and falling barometric pressure come before rain, and they *do* make damaged joints feel different. This allows some people with arthritis to predict changes in the weather. But that is about the only advantage I can think of to having arthritis, a disease affecting millions. While there is no known cure for arthritis, many people can find considerable relief by following the seven-point Cope with Arthritis Plan.

What part of the body is affected?
Arthritis involves damage to the joints, the parts of your body that allow you to bend. A "typical joint" is made of two bones whose ends fit together. So that the bones don't scrape and damage each other, the ends are covered with cartilage. (You have seen cartilage, or "gristle," at the end of a chicken drumstick.) The ends of the two bones are held together by a tough fibrous capsule which is lined by the synovial membrane. This membrane pro-

duces a lubricating fluid that lets the joint bend more easily.

What is the most common form of arthritis?
Osteoarthritis, often called "wear and tear" arthritis, affects 37% of adults and a whopping 97% of people over 60. It seems that the years take their toil on joint cartilage. Gradually it chips and wears away. Then the ends of the bones may scrape against cartilage chips or against each other. These and other changes cause swelling and pain. Since the joints of the spine, hips, and knees bear the most weight, they are affected most often.

As osteoarthritis develops, you may first notice pain in your fingers, backbone, hips, or knees. With many people, it hurts more in the morning. Stiffness, changes in your posture, and tiring easily are other signs. At an initial medical exam, a doctor will probably look you over, take X-rays, do blood tests, and have you move your joints around.

What is Rheumatoid Arthritis?
Also called rheumatism, this is the most crippling form of arthritis. It hits women three times as often as men, and usually shows up first between the ages of 20 and 50. Rheumatoid arthritis usually affects many joints, particularly in the hands and fingers. It can cause damage to the joint lining, destroy bones, and lead to deformities. Besides having joint pain, the person with rheumatoid arthritis may feel weak, stiff, feverish, and depressed, and may have a

1. Diet

Extra weight puts extra strain on the knees, hips, spine, and other joints. A safe reducing diet to get your weight into the normal range will relieve some pain. To start losing weight, cut down on sweets and alcohol, eat nutritious food, and stop eating just before you are full.

According to The Arthritis Foundation and most physicians, there are no special foods or vitamins that will help you cope with arthritis.
poor appetite. Rheumatoid arthritis tends to come (have "active periods") and go (have "periods of remission").

Checking for this disease, a doctor will often use X-ray, blood tests, and urine tests.

Are there other types of arthritis?
Yes, more than 100, including gout, ankylosing spondylitis, bursitis, and fibrositis. Arthritis is actually a broad category of diseases involving inflamed joints. The Cope with Arthritis Plan is geared to the two most common varieties, osteoarthritis and rheumatoid arthritis.

What is the Cope with Arthritis Plan?
The Plan is a common sense approach, calculated to give you relief from pain and appreciation for life's pleasures. If you have arthritis, I suggest you show this Plan to your doctor and figure out how to make it work for you.

2. Exercise

A good physical fitness program helps you deal with arthritis in three ways.

First, loosening up exercises keep your joints more flexible. Let's say you have a little arthritis in your spine. It becomes uncomfortable to bend, so you bend less. Your muscles and ligaments tighten up and you feel stiffer. Gentle stretching exercises, though, keep those muscles and ligaments looser and your back more comfortable. The same goes for hips, fingers, and all other joints.

Many people do well exercising in the morning to loosen up for the day and late in the evening to relax for sleep. Some find it easier when they take their aspirin or other medication twenty minutes before exercising.

The second way exercise helps is by strengthening your muscles. When your abdominal and back muscles are stronger, for example, they take some of the pressure off your spine. Swimming in a relaxed manner is an excellent way to take the weight off your joints, while you stretch and strengthen all your muscles.

Third, exercise improves your health, energy level, and mood in general, making it easier to take the arthritis in stride. A side benefit of exercise may be discovering ways you can position yourself and move comfortably for having sex.

3. Rest

If you have osteoarthritis, you may need extra rest. Gentle exercises, medication, a hot bath, or a bedtime massage may help you relax at bedtime.

If you have rheumatoid arthritis and it is "acting up," you will probably need lots of extra rest. Your doctor will probably advise you to stop your exercises and massage until the disease is back in remission.

A very firm mattress on top of a bedboard made of 1/2-inch thick plywood provides good support, allowing your back to relax in its natural position. When you lie down, imagine every muscle and joint relaxing and sinking into the mattress. Take a few nice deep yawns, and relax more each time you breathe out. *(See Chapter 4)*. You may find you feel better if you rest in bed for twenty minutes in the middle of the afternoon.

Rheumatoid arthritis often starts or flares up when a person is upset, run down, or overworking. Being happier and staying relaxed is part of both prevention and treatment. Various people may get great relief from meditation, prayer, deep breathing, biofeedback, or visualization exercises.

4. Heat

Years ago, my grandparents would treat themselves to the Russian steam baths on Coney Island. I enjoy the steam bath myself, especially in the win-

5. Massage

We all need to be touched, but massage is something more than that. It is something that a friend, a relative, a masseur or masseuse, or a physical therapist can do to help you relax. Muscles that have tightened to support sore joints like to be squeezed and stroked. For working on the back of a friend of yours, it is good to use the fingertips of both hands and press firmly on both sides of your friend's spine. It is also good to press and squeeze around the shoulder blades. In Chapter 22 of this book you will find instructions for a good head-neck-shoulder massage.

Massage should feel good. If it is painful, stop. Certain arthritic joints are too tender to be rubbed. ter, and have talked to many people with arthritis who like it. Heat, especially moist heat, is very relaxing to joints and muscles, although anyone in frail health or with a heart condition should check with a doctor before going to the steam bath.

A similar sort of relief is available at home by soaking in a hot tub for fifteen minutes. Some people hop into the tub as soon as they wake up and find it helps them loosen up quickly and face the day.

Heating pads can feel good, placed on sore muscles or joints. But be sure you get your doctor's instructions on how long to keep the pad on. And do not fall asleep on a hot pad!

Unless you have specific instructions from your physician, do not massage during flareups of rheumatoid arthritis.

6. Home Arrangements

Some people have arthritis to the point where they have trouble doing simple things around the house. Reaching low for kitchen utensils, high for pots and pans, is difficult for them. Cooking becomes easier when they set up their kitchens with everything at easy-to-reach levels. Shelves and peg boards are helpful.

If you have trouble keeping your balance while walking, avoid waxed floors or throwrugs. Instead, tacked down carpeting will give you some traction. Handrails can be installed in your shower and by the toilet. If you run into other household problems, an imaginative handyman can help you work out sensible improvements.

7. Medications

For many people with arthritis, following the first six points of this Plan will keep them quite comfortable. Others may also require medications.

Aspirin is the most common, the least expensive, and one of the most effective drugs to relieve pain and swelling. It is easier on the stomach when crushed and taken with food. It is cheaper, and just as effective, to purchase an inexpensive "house brand" at a drugstore. "Arthritis strength" aspirin products are simply larger tablets. Three regular aspirin tablets cost less than, and provide the same relief as, two "arthritis strength" tablets.

People with rheumatoid arthritis may be surprised at their doctors' advice to take aspirin even when they do not feel pain. This practice may be helpful in keeping joint swelling to a minimum and cut down on painful flareups.

Some people with osteoarthritis or rheumatoid arthritis cannot tolerate large amounts of aspirin. Others find that it does not provide the relief they need. Their doctors may turn to prescription medications such as indomethacin, phenylbutazone, gold salts, ibuprofen, and hydrocortisone. Each of them may reduce pain and swelling, and may also cause unpleasant — sometimes very serious — side effects. Unless your doctor directs otherwise, no aspirin should be taken at the same time as these prescription arthritis drugs. As with all medications, let your doctor know how you find the drug affects you.

Remember, medication is not a magic cure-all. It is one tool that can be used. If diet, exercise, rest, heat, massage, and home arrangements are all you need to Cope with Arthritis, more power to you!

For additional information on arthritis or referral to medical specialists, contact:

The Arthritis Foundation
National Office
475 Riverside Drive
New York, N. Y. 10027

For one approach to exercise as treatment, see *Pain-Free Arthritis,* by Dvera Berson. New York: Simon and Schuster, 1978, 96 pp., $6.95.

CARING FOR YOUR TEETH, GUMS, AND DENTURES

by Marsha Pike Palmer, R. D. H

Often we underestimate the connection between a healthy mouth and a healthy body, and think of dental health only in terms of teeth, cavities and dentures. Yet we also use our mouths for eating, speaking, swallowing and making facial expressions like smiling, and dental problems affect all of these functions. A disease in the mouth can cause headache or stomach ache, just as poor nutrition can cause dental problems. A better understanding of your dental health will help you take care of your teeth or dentures, prevent future dental problems, and make good use of the dental health team — dentist, dental hygienist, dental assistant, and dental laboratory technician. Here are answers to the questions my patients have most often asked me during my eight years' practice as a dental hygienist.

Does My Mouth Look Healthy?

Have you taken a good, deep look inside your own mouth lately? Get a mirror, pull back your lips, and analyze what you see.

77

Your teeth should be clean and white, free of food particles or stains. Any holes in your teeth, broken fillings, or empty spaces where teeth used to be should be brought to your dentist's attention. Yellowish stains may be due to nicotine in cigarette smoke, coffee or tea. Healthy teeth are important for tearing and grinding food, improving digestion and nutrition, and looking attractive.

Next, examine your gums, the soft tissue surrounding each tooth and protecting the jawbone. They should be pink in white people and have a brownish pigment in black people, be firm and hug each tooth like a snug collar around the neck. Are your gums red, swollen, sore, or bleeding easily? If so, you may have gingivitis, the first stage of gum disease. Almost every adult has some degree of gum disease, also called periodontal disease or pyorrhea. If it is not stopped, it affects the bone supporting the teeth and eventually the teeth loosen. Gum disease is responsible for about 80% of all teeth lost by adults.

Your use your tongue for tasting, chewing, swallowing, and speaking. How does it look? Your tongue should be clean and free from any coating or discoloration. The roof and floor of the mouth and the inside cheeks are all necessary for chewing, swallowing and speaking. The skin inside the mouth and cheeks should be smooth and pink (or brownish) and free from sores or white spots.

How does your breath smell? A strong odor may be caused by eating onions or garlic or by not brushing often enough. But constant bad breath may be a sign of tooth decay, gum disease or digestion problems.

Are There Mouth Diseases That Haven't Been Mentioned Yet?

Besides cavities and gum disease, it's important to know about *oral cancer*. It is similar to other malignancies and can affect the lips or any part inside the mouth. Oral cancer shows up first as a growth, a sore that does not heal, or a change in the mouth's color and texture. Pain may not be experienced until later stages. If any suspicious changes are noticed, a dentist should be consulted *at once*. Untreated oral cancer can cause disfigurement and, in advanced stages, even death. If detected early, it can be cured.

You can reduce your chances of developing oral cancer by avoiding chronic irritations, ill-fitting dentures, smoking, broken fillings of teeth, and excessive use of alcohol. Over-exposure to the sun may cause cancer of the lip.

What Can I Do To Keep My Mouth Healthy?

Your natural teeth, if you still have all or some of them, could last the rest of your life. It is important to see your dentist at least once or twice a year for diagnosis and treatment of the three diseases mentioned above, and for a professional cleaning. Diseased teeth should be repaired whenever possible. If some teeth are too damaged to save, it is important to have them removed to end the spread of infection. When these problems are taken care of, you can keep your mouth clean and control the formation of dental plaque.

What is Dental Plaque?

Plaque is a sticky film that forms constantly on your teeth. At first, it may be invisible, but with time it collects bacteria ("germs") and food. The bacteria can act on sugar in the food to produce acids. These acids attack tooth enamel, thus starting cavities. Plaque forms both above and below the gumline and can develop into hard deposits, called calculus or tartar, which irritate the gums. Calculus must be removed by a professional. But with regular brushing and flossing you can remove most of the film, bacteria, and food debris from your mouth before it hardens.

What is the Best Way to Brush?

Start with a good *soft* toothbrush. (A soft electric brush may be easier to handle for some people, including those with extreme arthritis of the hand or those weakened by strokes.) Many dentists recommend a brush with a straight handle, flat brushing surface and nylon bristles.

Place the bristles where the teeth and gums meet, turned at an angle toward the gum. Move the brush gently but firmly from side to side with short strokes about half a tooth wide. This gentle wiggling removes the plaque and massages the gums. This massage improves circulation to your gums and exercises the tissue. Use the same method on the inside surface of the teeth (the tongue side). Also brush the chewing surface to remove food debris in the grooves. A thorough brushing should be done at least once a day. Your dentist or dental hygienist may have additional suggestions for your particular mouth.

Toothpaste may leave a fresh clean taste in the mouth, but a dab of baking soda on your brush, an inexpensive "old-fashioned" method, cleans your teeth just as well. Many toothpastes have fluoride added to make the tooth structure more resistant to decay. Fluoride is also found in most city water supplies, or it can be applied in the dental office.

What About Dental Floss?

Flossing once a day is as important as brushing. You can get dental floss, a special waxed or unwaxed thread, at most drug stores and supermarkets. It helps clean between your teeth and gently massages your gums. Here's a good technique:

Take a piece of floss about 18 inches long and wrap most of it around one of your middle fingers. Wind the rest around the same finger on your other hand. As you floss, wind the used parts onto your second hand.

Use your thumbs and forefingers to guide the floss, with about an inch between your hands. Hold the floss tightly and use a *gentle* back and forth motion to get it between two teeth. Be careful not to let it snap into the gums.

When the floss reaches the gum, wrap it around the curve of the tooth and slide it under the gum until you meet a little resistance. Then hold the floss against the tooth and move it back and forth against the side of the tooth. Now stay between the same two teeth and clean between the other tooth and gum. Continue around the mouth, cleaning each tooth and gum and between all teeth at the contacts. This will take about five minutes. You may need some practice in front of a mirror to get the knack. Ask your hygienist for help if you need it.

Should I Use a Mouthwash?

Mouthwashes have no proven medical value such as "killing germs," though they may make your mouth feel fresh. For a good, inexpensive rinse, try salt water (1 teaspoon salt in 8 ounces of warm water). Gargling with warm salt water also helps soothe a sore throat.

What About Tooth Decay?

A sensitivity to sweets may signal a cavity forming. However, you can't feel most cavities until they are very deep. Regular examination with x-rays will detect cavities at an early stage. The dentist can then remove the decay and insert a filling before you are in pain. A silver amalgam filling is used if the cavity is small. When the cavity is large, a gold filling (inlay, onlay, or crown) may be necessary to support the tooth. White filling material and white caps are available for repairing front teeth where metal would show.

A decayed tooth cannot repair itself. Unless treatment is provided, decay proceeds through the enamel and all the way into the pulp — the vital center of the tooth where the nerves and blood vessels are. When the decay enters the pulp, an infection occurs and an abscess at the end of the root may develop. This may be acutely painful.

Deep decay or an accidental blow may damage the pulp of the tooth. Often such a tooth can be saved by root canal treatments involving removal of the damaged pulp and placing suitable filling inside the tooth.

What If Some Teeth Cannot Be Saved?

Some teeth cannot be repaired and must be removed (extracted). Missing teeth should be replaced, since each tooth depends on the next for stability, and spaces between teeth weaken the gums and bone support.

Lost teeth can be replaced in several ways. In many cases, a fixed bridge can be made. This entails making caps or crowns on the teeth on either side of the open space, suspending an artificial tooth in the space, and cementing the whole unit in the mouth. Your dentist can provide special cleaning instructions important to maintain the bridge.

A partial denture can be made when several upper or lower teeth are missing. Partials, as they are called, can be removed for cleaning and should be brushed with a regular brush and toothpaste to remove plaque accumulations. If you lose all of your upper or lower teeth, full dentures may be necessary. If you are losing your lower teeth, ask your dentist if a few of these teeth can be saved. A partial lower denture is usually much more comfortable than a full lower denture.

Before teeth are removed, you and your dentist should discuss your case. You may want to consider an immediate denture, placing temporary teeth in your mouth on the day of the extraction. This gives you some teeth during the healing process and will make you feel more comfortable socially. After the healing period, your dentist will take the final impression and the denture can be made.

In addition to extractions, changes in the bony ridge or gum tissue may be needed to provide adequate shape and tissue tone for denture support.

How Will My Dentures Affect My Appearance, Speech and Eating?

To provide a more natural look, many dentists now design dentures with characteristics very much like your natural teeth. The sense of awkwardness about your new teeth should lessen as your cheeks, lips, and muscles relax around the dentures.

Since speech consists of a detailed set of movements within the mouth, any major change in your mouth, such as getting dentures, may affect the way you talk. If you have any initial speech problems, they should clear up in a few weeks if you practice reading aloud and talking in front of a mirror.

Several eating and chewing problems may be encountered by denture wearers. For example, artificial teeth do not tear food as well as natural teeth, so food should be cut into small pieces. Sometimes the denture may become dislodged while chewing. When this happens, close the mouth and swallow to reseat the denture. Although most people naturally chew on only one side, dentures are designed for chewing on both sides. If you chew on one side, they tip, so concentrate on spreading food to both sides of the mouth. Without your natural teeth, your grinding power is reduced, so you must chew your food longer and more carefully.

If you wear an upper denture, skin and taste buds are covered and your mouth loses some of its sensitivity to taste and touch. Add more seasonings if your food tastes a little bland, or warm it to bring out the flavor. And check that you remove all bones from chicken and fish.

It is best to remove your dentures after each eating and clean them thoroughly to remove food debris and plaque before irritation can start. To clean your dentures, you can choose from many available commercial denture cleansers, or use a regular toothbrush and toothpaste, baking soda, or ordinary bar soap.

If My Dentures Don't Fit Well, What Can I Do?

If your dentures do not fit properly, see your dentist. *Do not adjust or repair your dentures yourself.* Periodically they will need to be relined (refit to your bony ridge). Your dentist can do this for you. Again, it should not be attempted as a do-it-yourself project, as even small mistakes in adjustment can cause serious damage, including sore spots which could result in oral cancer or loss of the bony support. If your dentist fails to find anything wrong with the fit of your denture and it still feels loose, an adhesive paste or powder may be recommended for your comfort and confidence.

Your mouth constantly changes, but dentures stay the same. Even if you do not notice any problems with your dentures, have an examination by a dentist at least once a year.

One Last Question: Is There Anything Special I Should Eat?

The foods you eat affect your whole body, including your mouth. There are several specific ways that nutrition relates to dentistry: sugar, coarse foods, Vitamin C, and calcium.

Sugar consumed in coffee, sodas, and sweets is the most common source of tooth decay. The sugar sticks to the plaque on the teeth and bacteria can then start cavities. "But don't we need sugar for energy?" some people ask. Yes, but let the sugar we need come from good healthy foods like bread, fruits and vegetables.

Coarse foods like carrots, celery, apples and cucumbers rub against the teeth while you chew. This gives the gums a good massage and helps keep teeth clean by removing old foods. Although chewing the right foods can help keep the mouth clean, it does not take the place of brushing and flossing.

Vitamin C is needed every day to keep your gums healthy. If you don't get enough Vitamin C your gums may bleed easily. Oranges, grapefruit, tomatoes, and broccoli are good sources of this vitamin. Some dentists and nutritionists recommend a daily supplement of Vitamin C (50-100 mg.) for people who do not receive enough in their foods.

Calcium is needed throughout life for the normal functioning of the body. Older people should have a daily serving of milk or a milk product, sardines or other calcium-rich food so that calcium is not removed from bones (including jawbones) to maintain the normal level of calcium in your blood.

Good luck, happy chewing, and keep smiling!

THE EYES HAVE IT

by Robert Skeist, R. N.

When I was a teenager, my mother started joking that her arms were too short to hold the newspaper. Farsightedness, or presbyopia, may first reveal itself in this way or as a headache or tiredness following close work. Reading glasses or bifocals may be extremely useful for coping with this, one of several eye problems common to older people.

The eye is shaped like a ball with a round bump in front. Behind that bump — the cornea — lie the clear lens and the tiny muscles that can change the shape of the lens to focus on something near or on another object far away. Light bounces off objects, passes through the lens and through a thick fluid inside the eyeball that helps maintain the eye's shape. The light then hits the retina at the back of the eyeball, and a picture forms. Tear ducts produce fluid to keep the eye surface moist and clean. Movement of the eyeball as a whole is governed by six muscles attached to the outside of the eyeball like ropes on a sailboat: tighten this one to look to the right, that one to look to the left, up, down, or at a diagonal.

Difficulties in vision may be caused by changes in any one of the parts of the eye. My mother's far-sightedness, for example, was caused by a loss of elasticity in the eye lens.

When the normally clear lens gradually turns gray or milky white, it is called a *cataract*. Someone developing a cataract may first notice that objects seem a little distorted or appear to have halos of light around them. Looking in the mirror, the normally black pupil in the center of the eye will appear cloudy.

No one knows why cataracts form, although injury to or surgery performed on the eye apparently increases the risk of the condition developing. The only currently known treatment is surgery, conducted when the cataract has "ripened" to the extent that it interferes with reading, driving, or another vision function the person identifies as of great importance. This surgery, done under local anesthesia, is generally quite safe, uncomplicated, and successful. Over 90% of cataract operations result in improved vision, by removing the darkened lenses and replacing them with implanted lenses, contact lenses, or special eye glasses. The advantages and disadvantages of each of these types of lenses should be discussed with the physician involved.

Medication is generally sufficient to treat *glaucoma*, the other major eye problem associated with aging. Glaucoma involves the blockage of a little passageway for fluid, resulting in a build-up of pressure inside the eye. This may cause tired eyes, headaches on one side, blurred vision, or loss of peripheral (side) vision. However, people developing the most common type of glaucoma, known as open angle, often notice nothing wrong until a great deal of vision has been lost.

Many cases of blindness due to glaucoma can be prevented by early detection with tonometry. This simple test involves a small instrument placed briefly on the surface of the eye to measure the pressure inside the eye. Performed at physicians' offices and at some public health screenings, tonometry tests should be taken at least once every two years by anyone over age 35. If glaucoma is discovered, special eye drops called miotics may be prescribed for daily use. They will not correct damage that has been done, but can prevent the condition from worsening.

In some people the macula, or central area of the retina, degenerates, making it difficult to see straight ahead in daylight. This *macular degeneration* may interfere with watching television, reading, or seeing people clearly. It may be coped with, though not cured, by using magnifying lenses or high-intensity lamps.

What about those "black spiders", the small moving dark spots that some people see wherever they look? Also called *floaters*, they are caused by changes in the fluid inside the eye. If they appear rapidly or accompanied by flashes of light, they could indicate a detached retina. In such cases, immediate treatment is necessary. In the vast majority cases, however, they are harmless, and there is no known treatment.

We tend to take *tears* for granted. They keep our eyes comfortable by moistening the delicate surface of our eyes and washing away irritants. With aging, though, many people produce fewer tears. The resultant dryness may cause irritation to the sensitive cornea and may lead to the overproduction of watery tears which lack the proper chemical balance to soothe the eyes. To treat dry eyes or an overproduction of watery tears, doctors may prescribe special eye drops, "artificial tears", to be used several times daily. A special lubricating ointment may also be prescribed to use at bedtime.

Certain medications — including insulin, diazepam (Valium), corticosteroids, and pills for high blood pressure — may cause *blurry vision*. So may diseases such as high blood pressure, diabetes, hardening of the arteries, cataracts, and glaucoma. It is important, therefore, to describe your vision problems to your general physician and your medications and health status to your eye doctor. *Eyestrain* may also result from reading, sewing, and other close work, especially if done for long stretches of time without a break or under poor lighting.

When seeking professional care for your eyes, it is helpful to know the difference between various specialists. An *ophthalmologist* is a physician who has gone through medical school and then specialized in medical and surgical treatment of the eye. An *optometrist* is not a physician, but someone trained specifically for testing the eyes for defects of vision in order to prescribe corrective glasses. An *optician*, also not a physician and not trained to diagnose medical problems, makes or sells eyeglasses, contact lenses, and other optical goods.

In addition to seeking appropriate professional help, there are some things that you yourself can do to help your eyes. The following exercises may help preserve your side vision and keep your eyes moist and relaxed. For anyone with eyestrain, I recommend them daily. It may be more relaxing to have a friend read you the instructions as you do them the first few times.

1. Sit down, take full breath, and relax. Close your eyes and see black. Feel your eyes and eyelids very relaxed. Move your shoulders easily, reach with your arms, and do gentle head circles. Feel your eyes grow moister. Blink slowly three times, and feel your eyelids spread tears across your eyes.

2. Hold your head still and relaxed. Slowly open your eyes. Without moving your head and without straining your eyes, look slowly as far as you can to the right. Notice how much you can see. Now very slowly look back in front of you and then all the way to your left. Do this exercise two more times, then close your eyes and relax.

3. Using the same approach, open your eyes and slowly look all the way up and all the way down three times. Now close your eyes and relax.

4. This time look across the long diagonal, from all the way on your upper right to way down at your lower left, then up to the right again. Do this easily, three times, and then do the same thing from the upper left to the lower right and back. Close your eyes and relax.

5. This last exercise is good for your eye lenses and the tiny muscles that hold them in place. If you are doing a lot of reading, typing, sewing, or any other sort of close work, it is good to do this one every half hour.

Look out a window at the sky and feel your eyes become very relaxed. Blink whenever you feel like it. Slowly look toward a faraway building, then at the window frame, and then at your own body. Look out at the sky. Close your eyes. Relax. Appreciate the miracle of vision.

For a catalogue of Large Print books, ask your Librarian or write to:
> Oscar B. Stiskin
> P. O. Box 3055
> Stamford, Connecticut 16905.

Free large-type booklets on health and medications are available from:
> Food and Drug Administration
> HFJ-10
> Rockville, Maryland 20857

For a variety of pamphlets on eyesight, contact:
> Better Vision Institute, Inc.
> 230 Park Avenue
> New York, N. Y. 10017

>> or

> National Society to Prevent Blindness
> 79 Madison Avenue
> New York, N. Y. 10016

I HEAR YOU!
HEARING CHANGES, HEARING AIDS

by Robert Skeist, R. N.

	True	False
1. I frequently ask that words or phrases be repeated.	___	___
2. It is difficult for me to hear when my back is turned to the speaker.	___	___
3. I strain to hear, or habitually turn one ear toward the speaker.	___	___
4. I have more trouble hearing and understanding conversation than someone with normal hearing.	___	___
5. It is extremely difficult or impossible for me to hear a faucet dripping in the room I am in.	___	___

If you checked "True" for any of these statements, have your hearing tested. That's the advice of the Chicago Hearing Society and its director, Dr. William Plotkin.

We use our hearing for conversation. We use our hearing to enjoy life, as when we appreciate music. We use our hearing to know what is happening around us — dogs barking, children playing, machines functioning, cars coming.

With aging, many of us notice hearing changes. "What did you say?" Frequently these words are the first sign of a hearing problem that makes conversation slower and more difficult. If the hearing gets worse, conversation becomes almost impossible, and isolation and loneliness may follow. As traffic and shouts grow harder to hear, the world becomes less predictable, more dangerous.

Approximately 14.5 million people in the U. S. have hearing problems, with older people affected more frequently than the young, and men more frequently than women. Some hearing problems are caused by build-ups of ear wax, ear infections, tumors, or drug side effects. These conditions can often be corrected, allowing the hearing to return to normal.

For older people, however, the most common cause of poor hearing is damage to the nerves in the inner ear that lead to the brain or damage to the part of the brain that receives and interprets sounds. A person with such nerve damage has trouble hearing soft sounds and high pitches. He or she may find loud sounds very annoying and may be bothered by humming or buzzing sounds in the ears. People who have lived in noisy cities or worked in noisy factories are more likely to develop these problems.

For most people with hearing loss due to nerve damage, there is no known cure. But hearing aids help millions of people. They work as sound systems, with microphones to make voices and all sounds louder.

The Chicago Hearing Society offers this advice about buying hearing aids:

1. **Start with a doctor's exam.** According to the U. S. Department of Health, Education and Welfare, each year thousands of people buy hearing aids who don't need them, receive no benefit from them, or would be helped more by medical or surgical treatment. Only after a professional examination can you know the cause of your hearing problem and whether it can be corrected.

2. **Ask your doctor where to go for the best possible hearing test.** Professionally trained people called audiologists are expert at this type of testing and will advise you on whether you can benefit from a hearing aid.

3. **Shop carefully.** If you do need a hearing aid, go to a good dealer, one who will not rush you into buying an aid. Do not let yourself be rushed. A hearing aid dealer must, by law, give you a brochure to read before you buy an aid. Many dealers will let you rent an aid to try it out for 30 days before you buy.

4. **Learn about your hearing aid.** It will *not* give you normal hearing again. It magnifies all sounds, not just conversation, so you will have to learn to "tune out" some of the background noises. Squealing is usually caused by a hearing aid that is too strong, does not fit right, or is not in place.

If you have a hearing problem, there are several other ways you can make your life easier. For example, you can have the telephone company install a telephone amplifier. Watching people's lips, facial expressions, and body movements as they talk makes it easier to understand them. Conversations are easier to understand indoors. You will hear more clearly when standing or sitting than when lying down (though there is a time and a place for everything). Many people are helped dramatically by learning to read lips.

What if your hearing is fine, and you are reading this chapter because a friend of yours is hard of hearing? Do not call from across the room to get your friend's attention. Come close and touch her, or say her name. Do not shout, but talk in a normal or *slightly* louder than normal voice. Speaking in deeper tones, talking a little more slowly than you usually do, and facing your friend will make your speech easier to understand. If you are not understood, re-word the sentence.

For additional reading, see:

Paying Through the Ear, an expose of the hearing aid industry available through the Gray Panthers National Office, 3635 Chestnut Street, Philadelphia, Pennsylvania 19104.

Pamphlets on hearing and hearing problems are available from:

> Public Affairs Committee, Inc.
> 381 Park Avenue South
> New York, N. Y. 10016

and from:

> Chicago Hearing Society
> 6 E. Monroe, 7th Floor
> Chicago, Ill. 60603

BE GOOD TO YOUR FEET!
by Robert Skeist R. N.
and
Leonard Winston, D. P. M.

Our poor feet! We consider them ugly or funny-looking, stuff them into poor-fitting shoes, and work them all day long. We seldom do daily foot care or get help for minor problems. Then we complain about the trouble our feet give us!

It is time we appreciate the marvelous construction of the foot, a complex assembly of twenty-six bones moved by seventeen muscles. Time we appreciate the amazing task the feet perform, making contact between our bodies and the earth for balance and movement. Time we learn how to prevent many foot problems, how to react to problems that do develop, how to make our feet feel good.

Use your feet. Walk! Walking is a mild, enjoyable form of exercise. It can postpone and perhaps prevent the development of the disabilities usually associated with aging, including heart disease and depression.

Buy a good pair of running shoes for flexibility and comfort. When you begin, walk briskly for just

15 minutes or so each day. To make it more enjoyable, get a friend to join you. After a week or two, increase your level of activity a little bit each day. Soon you will be walking half an hour a day.

If your feet ache a little when you get home, rinse them in cold water. Then sit back in a comfortable chair or lie in bed for five or ten minutes with your feet up. This relaxes them and lets the blood flow easily back to your heart.

Ready, set, wiggle! Walking is great exercise, but each time a 125-pound woman takes a step, she places 250 pounds of pressure on her foot. Day after day, she is on her feet, and they get sore. This woman may be familiar with exercises for her back, her neck, or her legs. But what about exercises for feet? Here are some that will help relax and invigorate them after a walk or any time of day:

To start, remove your shoes and socks, make yourself comfortable in your chair, and wiggle your toes in every conceivable way. Point your toes away from you and feel a stretch across the top of your foot all the way up to your knee. Then point your toes up and toward your face until you feel a stretch from your heel all the way up the back of your leg. Repeat this stretch five times.

To get at another set of muscles, turn your feet in circles around your ankles. Pretend you have a pen between your toes and you are drawing big circles with your toes. Make these circles five times in each direction.

Third, imagine your floor is covered with marbles. With one foot at a time, grab as many marbles as you can with your toes. If you have trouble picturing this, recall the last time you were at a zoo and saw apes or monkeys using their feet to pick up choice carrots or raw onions off the floors of their cages. Pick up your imaginary marbles five times with each foot, feeling the stretch through your entire foot.

Shop carefully for shoes. Corns, calluses, bunions, and sore feet are often caused by shoes that are too tight. It helps to shop in the afternoon, when your feet are larger, and to wear the kind of socks or stockings you plan to use with your new shoes. Don't automatically buy the same size shoe each time, since the man who takes a size 9½ in one shoe may need a 10 in another style.

Because one foot is often larger than the other, try on both shoes and choose a pair that fit your larger foot. Now stand up and check to see that you have a least half an inch to spare in the toes and that the shoes are comfortable at the widest part of your foot.

Laced up shoes give the best support. We recommend soft leather oxfords with leather soles and heels no more than half an inch to one inch high.

For a person with calluses, a shoe with a thicker sole may be considerably more comfortable.

What about socks? Heavy white cotton or wool socks may not be considered the height of fashion in all circles, but they are the best for the health of your feet. They cushion your feet as you walk, absorb sweat, and are free of irritating dyes. Socks should be changed every day. Loose woolen socks may be worn at night to keep your feel warm.

Many women prefer to wear nylons. While some have no problems with these stockings, others find that their feet become sweaty, smelly, or itchy, especially in hot weather. A compromise between style and health is available in the form of stockings with cotton bottoms and nylon tops.

Circular elastic garters and tight elastic-top hose may cut off your circulation, so never wear them. Your doctor may recommend special support stockings. These help the blood return from your feet to your heart, reduce leg strain, and reduce the risk of blood clots. If you use them, put them on safely and effectively. First sit or lie for ten minutes with your legs up on a chair or a cushion to drain the blood away from your feet and calves. Then put on the stockings and smooth away any folds or wrinkles.

Consider shoe inserts. If you have weak arches or "flat feet," a pair of arch supports or "orthotics" provided by a podiatrist might make your walking more comfortable. Made especially to fit your feet and placed inside of shoes, they support your arches. This helps you walk in a way that takes some pressure off of sore ankles, knees, and hips.

Cut your toenails straight across. A lot of people find it tempting to cut their nails round, or pick at them until all of the "white part" is gone. This can lead to ingrown toenails that may dig into skin, hurt, and require treatment by your podiatrist or physician. It is best to cut your nails straight across, then use a file on the rough edges.

Let your feet enjoy a bath. This is especially important for people with diabetes or poor circulation. Bathe your feet daily with lukewarm (**not** hot) water and mild soap. After a thorough rinsing, dry them gently, using a soft towel and a blotting technique. Pay special attention to the skin between your toes. If the skin is cracked there, you may have athlete's foot, a fungus infection. This can be treated with non-prescription creams and powders, and by cleaning and drying between the toes twice a day.

If your feet are very sweaty and smelly, wash them twice a day and dry them completely. Next put on rubbing alcohol or witch hazel, let your feet dry, and sprinkle on some foot powder or talcum powder.

Dry, flaky feet need love. Extreme dryness can cause cracks, scaling, sores, and infections which call for the attention of a podiatrist. It is better to take care of your feet when you first notice they are dry. Soak them for ten minutes each day in warm water (about 95°F.). Dry them well, including between the toes, and massage in a non-perfumed lotion.

Do you have corns and calluses? They are caused by the building up of hard skin at points where shoes cause pressure. In general, they should be treated by a podiatrist, who may instruct you to rub them gently with a fine emery board or pumice stone or to apply petroleum jelly and cover with an adhesive bandage. Non-medicated corn pads may be useful to temporarily relieve pain. Never cut calluses or corns with a razor or knife or apply strong chemicals to your feet!

Live it up: massage your feet! Now that you are exercising and caring for your feet, it is time to add a special treat — foot massage. There are many techniques, and with experience you may develop your own style.

Start by washing your feet, patting them dry, wriggling and stretching them. Now use both hands on one foot and squeeze gently all over it. Take your thumbs and make firm circles all over the bottom of your foot, especially where you can feel that muscles are tight or sore. Pull your toes gently apart and lightly tug on each toe. Do the same with your other foot. Then soothingly rub in a little lotion or petroleum jelly.

Washing and massaging another person's feet, by the way, is a wonderful expression of friendship.

For additional reading:

On Your Feet by Elizabeth H. Roberts, D. P. M., Rodale Press, Emmaus, Pennsylvania, $8.95. A practicing podiatrist tells you how to maintain foot health and comfort from infancy to old age. With large type and clear illustrations.

Literature is also available from:

American Podiatry Association
Publications Section
20 Chevy Chase Circle, N. W.
Washington, D. C. 20015

BE OF STRONG HEART!
by Susan Nick, R. N.

Picture yourself pumping water at a steady rhythm into a rubber hose. About once a second you push down the handle and water rushes out, flowing with great force through the hose. As you lift up the handle, the water still flows, but less forcefully.

The pump is that indispensable muscle, your heart. The water is that precious fluid, your blood, carrying food, oxygen, and protection against infection to every cell of your body. The hose is a blood vessel. The force of the water pushing through the hose is the pressure of your blood flowing through your blood vessels, your blood pressure.

Lately an increasing number of people in their thirties and forties are being diagnosed with high blood pressure or heart disease. Among people in their sixties and older, problems with the "pump" and "hose" are the leading cause of death. The first part of *To Your Good Health* describes the basics of good health, including good diet, proper exercise, a sense of meaning, and sound sleep. At any age, these will help keep your heart strong and your blood pressure normal.

Many people, though, need more specific information about heart and blood vessel problems and how to avoid or respond to them.

High Blood Pressure

At your last medical appointment, your nurse probably took your blood pressure and mentioned something like "120 over 80" or "174 over 92." To get an idea of what these numbers mean, think of that pump and hose again. As you pump and release, the water pressure rises and falls, rises and falls. Similarly, with each beat of your heart your blood pushes forcefully against the arteries, then less forcefully. The first number in a blood pressure reading, called the systolic pressure, indicates your blood pressure as your heart pumps. The second number, called the diastolic pressure and always lower than the systolic, shows your blood pressure as your heart rests between pumps.

120/80 is often considered the "normal" blood pressure, just as 98.6° F. is considered the "normal" temperature. Actually, what is normal blood pressure varies from person to person. Perhaps your pressure for years has been around 140/84 and your best friend's has been around 114/66. If your pressure suddenly dropped as low as your friend's, you might feel very faint, while your friend would feel "normal." Your pressure also varies with the time of day — lower when you first wake up, higher as you start the day's activities, lower again in the evening. Exercise temporarily raises your blood pressure, which returns to a lower level when you rest. Emotional stress also raises blood pressure temporarily. For these reasons, your blood pressure in the course of a day may go, for example, from 130/76 to 152/82 to 138/74.

Physicians frequently define any person who consistently has a blood pressure of 160/90, or a higher stystolic or diastolic reading, as having high blood pressure. Hypertension, as this disease is also called, occurs in one out of every three people over the age of 50. Uncontrolled, it can lead to heart attacks, strokes, and severe kidney damage.

Some people react to high blood pressure by developing headaches, dizziness, fatigue, and shortness of breath. In a way, they are the lucky ones. For they realize that "something is wrong," and are likely to seek medical attention. But half of the hypertensives do not realize their condition. Frequently they do not feel any clear symptoms of the disease. This explains why high blood pressure has been nicknamed "The Silent Killer." It also explains why each of us should have our blood pressure checked at least once a year.

What can be done to prevent high blood pressure? First of all, avoid cigarette smoking. Second, keep your weight down, not with a crash diet but with a sensible program of good nutrition, based on your doctor's advice and the guidelines in Chapter 2.

It is particularly important to limit your intake of cholesterol, a fatty substance that can build up in your blood vessels and cause them to narrow and lose flexibility. It is not yet known if the buildup already present in an individual's blood vessels can be reduced, but it is possible and important to prevent further build-up. Here are some ways to reduce your cholesterol intake:

1. Have no more than three eggs per week.
2. Eat less shellfish and organ meats.
3. Choose fish, poultry, and veal instead of beef.
4. Trim the excess fat off meat before cooking it.
5. Broil foods instead of frying them.
6. Replace butter with margarine.
7. Replace whole milk, cheese and yogurt with low-fat dairy products.
8. Use vegetable oils labeled "poly-unsaturated."

Working with your physician, you can see how your blood cholesterol level reacts to this type of diet. Different people can tolerate different amounts of cholesterol.

Another dietary measure to help keep blood pressure down is cutting back on salt. Salt absorbs water — the more salt you consume, the more fluid your body retains. Excess fluid in the blood vessels raises your blood pressure and forces your heart to do more work. If you read the labels on the food products you buy, you will notice how salt or sodium is added to so many things. Snack foods and canned vegetables are particularly high in salt. Even over-the-counter drugs often contain sodium. You can take the salt shakers off your table and still get as much salt as your body needs from foods you eat every day.

Caffeine, too, can raise your blood pressure. Coffee, tea, cocoa, and cola drinks can be replaced with decaffeinated coffee, grain drinks or herbal teas, and juices.

Swimming, bicycling, and jogging are a few types of exercise that contribute to lower blood pressure. So does walking, as Chapter 1 describes. It makes sense to check with a physician familiar with various exercise approaches for help in deciding what type of activity is best for you.

Finally, relax. Constant emotional stress or physical nervousness raises blood pressure. Relaxing breathing, talking with a dear friend, gardening, and taking a pleasant walk are among the dozens of possible approaches to calming down.

Confronting these risks — smoking, obesity, stress, lack of exercise and intake of cholesterol, salt, and caffeine — is essential to both the prevention of high blood pressure and to its treatment. But sometimes additional treatment is necessary, and your doctor may prescribe medication. Anti-hypertensives lower blood pressure directly, while diuretics ("water pills") have a similar effect indirectly, by reducing the amount of excess fluid in the body. Everyone is different — if you and a friend both have hypertension, you may need different drugs.

It may be that your high blood pressure medication does a great job a reducing your blood pressure, but you feel dizzy when you get out of bed or up from a chair. This side effect is easy to control in moving slowly from lying to sitting, from sitting to standing. Depression, potassium imbalance, visual disturbances and sexual impotence are other possible reactions to medications. If you notice any new problems in yourself or a loved one, ask the physician involved to review the medications.

Coronary Artery Disease

Coronary arteries are vessels which bring oxygen and nutrients to the heart so it can continue its pumping action. In a condition called atherosclerosis, fatty deposits harden and narrow these vessels, preventing enough blood from getting through. This is similar to the problem in your bathroom sink when the drain is clogged with hairs, except that you cannot reach into your blood vessels to clean them out.

When insufficient amounts of blood and oxygen reach your heart, a warning known as angina pectoris is triggered. Angina may be localized in the area of the heart, or it may radiate to the shoulder and left arm. These attacks often occur when a person is shovelling snow, lifting heavy objects, or rushing around. They are warnings to slow down and rest. Doctors often prescribe the medication nitroglycerine to relieve angina attacks. This medication is usually taken as a small pill which is dissolved under the tongue and usually brings relief in 3 to 5 minutes. Taking and storing nitroglycerine correctly requires special instructions from your doctor, nurse, or pharmacist.

Heart Attacks

Heart attacks are the number one killer in this country, causing 650,000 deaths each year. Your physician may speak of a coronary thrombosis, a coronary vascular occlusion, or a myocardial infarction. These all mean that the blood supply has not been able to get to all areas of the heart. A blockage in the arteries is usually caused by a clot that forms in the coronary artery or by a part of a clot that forms elsewhere, breaks off, and travels until it lodges in the heart. It may also be caused by the bursting of a tiny vessel due to high blood pressure. Where the blood supply has been cut off, the tissue dies from lack of oxygen and starts to form scar tissue. Though this usually occurs in only a tiny area of the heart, it may cause major problems.

The victim of a heart attack may experience a great deal of pain, often in the center or the left chest and in the left shoulder, arm and back. Some people feel the pain from the jaw down to the abdomen, and others feel tightness in their chest, like suffocation, along with sweating and nausea.

If you are with someone having a heart attack, use the telephone emergency number to call for medical halp. This will bring an ambulance with trained paramedics to help in treatment. If you are trained to give cardiopulmonary resuscitation (CPR) start it immediately. If you have not received any other training, help the heart attack victim by loosening tight clothing and washing his or her face and neck with a cool wet cloth. See that there is fresh air circulating, and stay with the person until the paramedics arrive.

Pacemakers

An incredible natural electrical system normally stimulates the heart muscle to pump enough times each minute to prcvide adequate blood circulation. If the number of beats per minute drops, it is sometimes necessary to implant a pacemaker.

In this procedure, a box smaller than a pack of cigarettes is placed under the skin just beneath the shoulder bone or in the upper abdomen. A wire connected to the box is threaded through a vein and into the heart. This battery-operated pack sends the electrical impulse along the wire to stimulate contractions of the heart. Like any battery, the one in a pacemaker runs down after a number of years and needs to be replaced. Since the pacemaker is implanted right under the skin, this is easily done.

Once the pacemaker is implanted and has healed virtually all activity can be resumed. Caution is required in the vicinity of a limited number of electrical appliances, including certain microwave ovens. When they are turned on, you should be 10-15 feet away from them if you have a pacemaker. People with pacemakers are taught to take their own pulse. This way they can monitor their pacemakers and, with a little help from technology, be of strong heart.

For related pamphlets, contact:
American Heart Association
Inquiries Section
7320 Greenville Avenue
Dallas, Texas 75231

For an educational poster and card, contact:
Metropolitan Life Insurance Company
Health and Safety Education Division
One Madison Avenue
New York, N. Y. 10010

CONTROLLING DIABETES

by Robert Skeist, R. N.

Diabetes affects an estimated 5,000,000 people in our country, 80% of them over 45 years old. Uncontrolled, it can cause great discomfort, circulation problems, blindness, and even death. But for the great majority of people diabetes can be controlled with a program including weight control, exercise, and a nutritious diet low in sweets.

The carbohydrates you eat as starches and sugars are broken down by your digestive system into simple sugar molecules called glucose. This glucose is carried by your bloodstream to every cell of your body to be burned as fuel. But without insulin, a hormone produced in the pancreas, glucose cannot move from your blood into your cells. If your pancreas produces no insulin, or not enough, you develop the symptoms of diabetes. Since not enough glucose is supplied as fuel to your cells, you become tired and weak. As too much glucose builds up in your blood stream, your kidneys do their best to filter it out and you urinate frequently. This leaves you short of water, extremely thirsty, and with dry, itchy skin.

All this time, your cells crave glucose. Since they are not getting it from your food, your body tries to fuel itself in another way. It breaks down fat molecules, releasing additional glucose into the blood along with ketones, leading to rapid weight loss and the development of a chemical imbalance called ketosis.

With your cells still unable to use the glucose in your bloodstream, your body tries one more futile approach: it breaks down protein, resulting in smaller muscles, lower resistance to infection, and slower healing. All this time, what your system desperately needs is to be put back into balance.

If you or a friend or family member note any of the symptoms described above, a medical examination is called for. The nurse or doctor will probably ask about your urination, thirst, hunger, strength, healing, diet, exercise, and the medical histories of members of your family. If diabetes is suspected, your urine and blood will probably be tested. The simplest test involves dipping a chemically-coated plastic or paper strip or dropping a tablet into a urine specimen and checking for a color change. For a more accurate test, the doctor or nurse may instruct you to go without food for several hours or take a special meal or drink, and then have blood drawn at specific intervals.

If diabetes is detected, diet is the first area of concern. Most adult diabetics are overweight, putting an extra strain on their bodies and making diabetes worse. Weight loss, then, is one essential goal. Also, carbohydrates must be chosen with care. It is helpful to eat large amounts of rice, other grains, and grain products.

These foods help your body stabilize the amounts of glucose and insulin in your blood. Simple carbohydrates such as table sugar, honey, and sweetened desserts may seriously strain your system and should simply be eliminated from diabetics' diets. Since diabetics face an increased risk of developing heart and blood vessel disease, it is especially important for them to cut down on saturated fats and cholesterol. (See Chapter 2.) Small meals spaced at regular intervals throughout the day also helps your body make better use of insulin.

Exercise is the next area to focus on. Walking, swimming, and other exercises that work the heart and lungs are helpful to burn off calories, reduce weight, and reduce the risk of cardiovascular disease. Exercise also helps your body make better use of whatever insulin it does produce.

For many, dietary and exercise changes are enough to keep their bodies in balance, but some diabetics need and are helped by medications. Those who produce no insulin of their own will need injections of insulin obtained from the pancreases of animals or produced in a laboratory. If this is true for you, be sure that your nurse or doctor teaches you the right way to give yourself shots. For those who produce some insulin, but not enough, oral hypoglycemics may be prescribed. These pills are not recommended as frequently now as in the past, since some of them have been implicated in cases of heart disease. Seeking an alternative to oral hypoglycemics, some diabetics have been motivated to control their disease by sticking more consistently to a program of good diet and exercise.

Day to Day

People with diabetes should clean their feet daily, dry them thoroughly, keep them soft with lotion, and check them for cuts or bruises. Toenails should be kept clean and smooth and cut straight across. Removal of corns, calluses or warts should not be attempted nor even minor foot surgery performed without special attention from an experienced physician or podiatrist.

Skin should be kept clean and dry and bruises that are slow to heal should be reported at once to the doctor. Teeth and gums should be brushed twice a day with a soft-bristle brush and carefully flossed daily. Mouth sores or bleeding gums should be reported to a dentist, and dentists should be immediately informed of patients with diabetes.

Like most diseases, diabetes is made worse by stress. Sleep, rest, relaxation, and a regular schedule will help keep your digestive system functioning smoothly and your energy level steady.

Finally, it helps for diabetics to learn how their bodies react to low blood sugar (hypoglycemia) and high blood sugar (hyperglycemia). Low blood sugar may be caused by taking too much insulin, skipping a meal or getting more exercise than usual. It often comes on suddenly and leads to a drunken appearance and behavior, hunger, and pale, wet skin. The immediate treatment is taking sugar, chocolate, or orange juice, or as your doctor prescribes.

High blood sugar may be caused by skipping a dose of medication, eating sweets or too big a meal, getting less exercise than usual, reacting to the stress of infection, or severe tension. Hyperglycemia often comes on more gradually than hypoglycemia and leads to thirst, drowsiness, and flushed, dry skin. Untreated, either glucose/insulin imbalance may lead to coma and death. So learn to understand your body's signals, know what to do in an emergency, and - most important - keep your system in balance with medication (if prescribed), a healthy diet, and exercise. (*For travel advice for diabetics, see Chapter 16.*)

For free pamphlets on diabetes in English and Spanish, contact:

American Diabetes Association
600 Fifth Avenue
New York, N. Y. 10020

UP IN SMOKE
by Robert Skeist, R. N.

Death in the West is one of the best films you will never see. Produced by a British television crew in 1976, it focuses on the lives of six real-life American cowboys. These six are highly reminiscent of the rugged outdoor types featured in Marlboro's $30 million annual advertising campaign. The virile image must be a successful one, since two trillion Marlboros are sold annually in the United States.

At what price?

Five of the real-life cowboys in *Death in the West* have lung cancer. The sixth has emphysema. The cowboys' doctors, interviewed in the film, say that their patients' diseases were caused by heavy cigarette smoking.

Now add some dramatic background footage of the mountains of New Mexico and some dramatic "high noon" music, and you have quite an effective anti-smoking film. So effective that when Marlboro manufacturer Phillip Morris viewed the film on British television, they sued and won a court decision that bars any future showing of *Death in the West*.

Smoking dramatically increases the odds of suffering from lung cancer, emphysema, heart attack, and stroke. It also causes earlier wrinkling of the skin, weakens bones, reduces oxygen supply to the brain, yellows teeth, fouls breath, and leads to coughing and wheezing. Smoking makes it harder to walk, to feel emotion, to make love. And it could easily run you $500 annually — a lot of money up in smoke.

Why, then, do so many people find it difficult to stop smoking? For one thing, nicotine is addictive. Yes, addictive, as alcohol is or barbiturates are. Withdrawal from nicotine creates a physical and emotional craving for more smoking. Secondly, smoking gives people "something to do", provides some oral satisfaction, and subdues feelings of anxiety. In addition, powerful interests push us to smoke. U. S. retail sales of tobacco products in 1978 totalled $17 billion, equal to the Gross National Product of Greece. No exception to the rule that successful corporations have friends in Congress, tobacco producers win politicians' favor by making sizable campaign contributions through the Tobacco People's Public Affairs Committee. This helps assure that each anti-smoking government dollar is far outweighed by subsidies to grow more tobacco.

In recent years we have seen the growth of an array of devices and clinics to help people stop smoking. One government brochure suggests a variety of techniques including switching to a brand you hate, chewing toothpicks, drinking lots of water, exercising, and deep breathing.

Recent studies indicate that stopping smoking at any age initiates efforts by the body to repair the damage. Disease risk then decreases and breathing improves. The effort to stop smoking is worth it, because you are.

For further information, write for "Clearing the Air, A Guide to Quitting Smoking." DHEW Publication No. (NIH) 79-1647, Office of Cancer Communications, National Cancer Institute, Bethesda, Maryland 20019.

For pamphlets, films, and speakers, about smoking, contact:

> American Cancer Society
> Public Education Department
> 777 Third Avenue
> New York, N. Y. 10017

For information about the fight for non-smokers' rights, exposés of the tobacco industry, and anti-smoking posters and buttons, contact:

> ASH — Action on Smoking and Health
> 2000 H Street, N. W.
> Washington, D. C. 20006

CANCER
REDUCING YOUR RISK
by Robert Skeist, R. N.

A few people muttered their disapproval. Two women were so uncomfortable that they left the room in the middle of my talk. I was addressing a Chicago senior citizens' club on behalf of the Seniors' Health Program of Augustana Hospital. My fellow nurses and I had spoken to that club two dozen times before on topics such as medications, arthritis, nutrition, exercise, and blood pressure. Never before had anyone walked out on us. But never before had our topic been cancer.

Cancer, that's the word, the subject that made those people feel so uneasy. It scares us all. It reminds us of newspaper articles about the dangers of hot dogs and saccharine, of the nuclear reactor accident at Three Mile Island in Pennsylvania, of serious chemical and surgical treatments. It reminds us of the deaths of people dear to us and of our own vulnerability.

But working individually and together, we can greatly cut down the risk of getting cancer. It is for that reason, for the optimistic side of the story, that

I took the chance of making a few members of that club uncomfortable. For the same reason, most of those who stayed told me they were grateful for the information.

The Seven Warning Signs

A good place to start learning about cancer is with the seven warning signs — clues the body gives that a malignancy may be developing. These symptoms could be caused by conditions far less serious than cancer, but why take a chance? Any one of these warning signs should send you immediately to a qualified physician for an examination, since those cancers detected early are most easily cured.

1. Have your bowel movements or urination habits changed?

Constipation, gas pains, and rectal bleeding may be early signs of cancer of the colon. these same symptoms could also be caused by less serious dietary or stress problems. A thorough exam, including a proctoscopy (an examination of the inside of the large intestine using an instrument inserted through the anus) is part of the doctor's "detective work."

Many older men develop problems with their prostate glands. The donut-shaped prostate rests below the bladder and encircles the urethra, the tube through which the urine is passed. The prostate may grow too large, causing problems such as difficulty or pain when starting to urinate, frequent urination, or bloody urine. Pain in the lower back, pelvis, or upper thighs may come with the bargain. Most prostate conditions are benign (that is, not cancerous) but some cases do involve cancer. Men, do not "just live with" difficult or bloody urination. See a doctor to have your condition thoroughly evaluated and treated.

2. Do you have a sore that will not heal?

Look inside your mouth or on your skin for any areas that are sore, raised, lumpy, or flaky.

3. Do you have any unusual bleeding or discharge?

Women after the menopause who pass blood through the vagina should go immediately for an examination. This bleeding could be an early sign of cancer of the uterus (the large round part of the womb). To check for early stages of cancer of the cervix (the narrow opening of the uterus) each woman should have the simple Pap test done once a year.

Another possible place to find blood is mixed in with the stools. This could be caused by hemorrhoids, but could also be a sign of cancer of the colon.

4. Did you find a lump in your breast or elsewhere?

It is important for women to examine their own breasts once a month for any suspicious-feeling lumps. You can learn how to check yourself from a doctor or nurse or at a women's health clinic. Many lumps are benign, but is the lump in your breast or on any other part of your body is malignant (cancerous), catching it early allows the best chance for successful treatment with minor surgery.

5. Do you have trouble digesting your food or swallowing?

Indigestion, stomach pain, nausea, reduced appetite, and difficulty swallowing may be signs of stomach or esophageal cancer.

6. Do you notice a change in a wart or mole?

Report any wart or mole that gets larger, soft and bloody, or just strange-looking.

7. Are you hoarse and coughing?

This could be from the irritation of smoking, which can contribute to lung cancer. A "lump in the throat" and sore neck could be a sign of cancer of the larynx ("voice box").

Remember, none of these signs means that you have cancer. They are clues, hints, warning signs that *something* is wrong. A good examination will probably give you the reassurance that your problem is fairly minor and can be left alone or treated by methods such as improving your diet or stopping smoking. But if tests show that you do have cancer, chances for a cure are much better the sooner treatment starts.

Four Ways To Reduce Your Risk

Now let's take a step back from cancer-detection to cancer-prevention. Here are six ways you can cut down your odds of ever having cancer:

1. *Stop smoking.* "Stop-smoking clinics" are a growing business these days, with good reason. A pack-a-day smoker is three times as likely as a non-smoker to get lung cancer. Smokers also have more cancer of the mouth, esophagus, larynx, and bladder.

Smoking low-tar cigarettes lowers the risk. Smoking marijuana, according to drug authority Ronald Gaetano, R. Ph., may be even more irritating to the lungs than smoking regular cigarettes.

Pipe and cigar smokers are less likely than rigarette smokers to get lung cancer as long as they do not inhale. They still risk more mouth, esophagus, and larynx cancer than non-smokers.

2. *Go easy on the alcohol.* A heavy consumption of alcohol leads to an increase in cancer of the mouth, esophagus, and liver. Those people who

smoke heavily and drink heavily are fifteen times as likely as non-smokers/non-drinkers to get cancer of the mouth or esophagus.

3. *Eat well.* Cut down on animal and dairy fat and on organ meats, especially liver. They tend to trap and concentrate cancer-causing chemicals. Also, eat fewer highly-processed foods such as bacon, hot dogs, salami, smoked fish, and soda pop.

4. *Guard against the sun.* Especially if you are fair skinned, use a sun screen lotion.

Working Together To Stop Cancer

There is a limit to what each of us alone can do to reduce the risk of getting cancer. Stopping smoking does not stop industrial pollution. Giving up hot dogs does not solve the problem of work-place toxins. We can do much more if we join together to work for political changes. Following the 1979 nuclear power accident at Three Mile Island in Pennsylvania, many of us are more aware of the radiation hazards of nuclear energy. We can support the demand that the highest nuclear safety standards be upheld and that the sun be used as a safe energy source. Pressing for stricter air and water pollution laws and enforcing the laws already on the books will also reduce our risk of getting cancer. Making these changes will require the long-term cooperation of a strong consumer movement willing to take on some very powerful industries.

To understand how bringing home a paycheck may be hazardous to your health, take a look at the asbestos industry. An eminent panel of cancer experts affiliated with the World Health Organization has made an astounding prediction: out of 1,000,000 Americans who once worked in asbestos manufacturing plants or still are employed, 200,000 will die of lung cancer and another 50,000 will die of mesothelioma (cancer of the abdominal lining) (Chicago Sun-Times, "The Working Wounded," 1978). Decades after scientific evidence had been published concerning the serious health risks of working with asbestos, the asbestos industry fought efforts to inform its workers and implement safety procedures. Businesses avoided the cost of safety measures and workers paid the price — widespread asbestosis (lung scarring) and cancer.

An important figure in the fight for workers' health is Samual S. Epstein, M. D. , Professor of Occupational and Environmental Medicine at the University of Illinois School of Public Health. In his recent book, *The Politics of Cancer,* Dr. Epstein lists other work-lated cancers: "Some plastics workers develop . . . cancers from exposure to vinyl chloride. Workers with nickel and chromium have high lung cancer rates. Dye workers have high rates of bladder cancer. Workers exposed to benzene have increased rates of leukemia." Frequently, companies and company doctors do their best to keep employees and unions ignorant of these dangers.

Some occupational-related cancers take as long as 20 to 35 years to develop. Therefore, even readers of this book who retired long ago from work in asbestos plants (or shipyard, construction, or building demolition, which often involved exposure to asbestos) or other high-risk jobs mentioned above should contact their doctors for examinations and their unions for information, and legal advice.

As Anthony Mazzocchi, vice president of the Oil, Chemical, and Atomic Workers International Union, puts it, "Ninety percent of the cancers are environmentally caused. We can conduct the best cancer prevention program going if we win the right to know and the right to act on our knowledge."

For further information:

The Politics of Cancer by Samuel S. Epstein, M. D., Sierra Club Books, San Francisco, California, $12.50. A leading professor of occupational and environmental medicine argues convincingly and with careful documentation that the overwhelming majority of all human cancers are environmentally induced or related — and thus preventable. He attacks industry and governmental agencies and calls for political action by union, medical, and environmentalist groups.

ASBESTOS
National Cancer Institute
Bethesda, Maryland 20014
Toll-free telephone: 800-638-6694
(in Maryland call 800-492-6600)

Cancer Information Service
U. S. Department of Health, Education, and Welfare
Call toll-free 800-638-6694, 8:00 A. M. —12:00 P. M., seven days a week. Offers support, information on current treatments, printed materials, and referral to local resources.

Office of Cancer Communication
National Cancer Institute
Bethesda, Maryland 20014

Provides publications on cancer ranging from a layperson's booklet on progress against cancer to reports of survival rates of patients for 48 specific types of the disease.

American Cancer Society
Public Education Department
777 Third Avenue
New York, N. Y. 10017

Provides publications, speakers, films about what the individual can do; very weak in terms of addressing the corporations' role in spreading cancer.

Make Today Count, Inc.
514 Tama Building
P. O. Box 303
Burlington, Iowa 52601

Provides information on support groups for cancer patients.

ACHES AND PAINS
by Susan Nick, R. N.

We all experience pain at times. It may be a headache, a backache, pain in the joints, a sore neck, a stomach ache, or heartburn, and we each respond in our own way. One person feels annoyed, another person feels self-pity, a third person feels it is finally time to see a doctor, a fourth relaxes in a hot bath.

Thirty-five billion dollars is spent each year in the United States on hospitalizations, health services, medications and loss of work-compensation due to pain. What kinds of pain are there? What causes pain? What can you do about pain?

Acute pain comes on suddenly and may go away after a short while. It can be a useful warning for you, and it can help your doctor figure out what is wrong with you. Acute pain may be a sign of an injury or disease that needs the attention of a physician. For example, a sharp pain the lower right section of your abdomen could be caused by appendicitis. Pain may be a signal for you that you are doing something too strenuous for your body. For example, a forty-five-year-old who goes out jogging for the first time in ten years may develop aching legs or even chest pain.

Sometimes the problem is one place and the pain is someplace else. This is called referred pain. For example, the heart is on the left side of the chest, but someone having a heart attack may feel pain in the left arm as well as the chest. This acute pain is useful if it served as a warning to you and as a diagnostic aid to your physician.

The way you describe your pain can help your doctor figure out what is going on in your body. When you hurt, ask yourself these questions:

- Exactly where is the pain located?
- Does it stay in one area or does it spread over a large area?
- Is it burning?
- Is it a dull ache or a sharp pain?
- Is it there all of the time or does it come and go?
- What time of day is it worse?
- Is this before or after meals?
- How long have you had this pain?
- Does the pain come when you are upset or angry?
- If so, what is stirring up these emotions?
- Have you found any way to make it hurt less?

Your answers to these questions give your doctor a very useful set of clues. Then he or she has an easier job figuring out what is causing your acute pain

Chronic pain lasts a long time. It may not be present every minute, but comes back month after month, year after year. Once you and your doctor know what is causing the pain, it has no little value. You hear about this kind of pain from people with arthritis, migraine headaches, or unhealed ulcers.

Each of us reacts to pain differently. Sometimes this has to do with ethnic background and sex. Japanese men may bear their pain stoically and seldom complain. Latin American women, in contrast, may easily express their feeling of pain. Cultural influences can change over time. Not too many years ago American men thought it was a sign of weakness to cry. When they hurt, they "took it like men." Now it is more accepted in this country for men to show pain or sorrow with tears.

Specific childhood experiences may play a role in our reaction to pain as adults. Take the example of a young boy who gets special attention from his parents when he is sick. He gets presents, special treats to eat, or a lot more time together with Mom and Dad. This feels good. Then the boy grows up and finds his job getting tough or his family criticizing him. He may complain about pain to get other people to take care of him.

Meanwhile, a little girl scrapes her leg when jumping the neighbor's fence and her mother yells at her. She teases a dog, is bitten, and gets yelled at again. Her adult reaction to pain may be to hold it in so she is not criticized. What can you remember from your childhood about how you felt, and what your parents did when you felt pain?

Relieving Pain

The first thing many people do to relieve pain is turn to their medicine cabinets. What they find there will not treat the cause of the pain, but it may relieve the symptoms.

The most frequently used medications are those that are sold over-the-counter, without prescriptions. Aspirin is the main product in this non-addicting group. It is inexpensive and very effective for a wide range of symptoms. It reduces pain, fever and inflammation.

Codeine is a widely used, weak narcotic pain reliever. It is not addictive when used for limited periods of time in the amounts doctors prescribe. It is often used in combination with aspirin or aceta-mionophen (Tylenol, for example). These combination medications are sold only by prescription from your physician.

Narcotics, such as Morphine and Percodan, are highly addictive and should be used only when pain relief has not been achieved with milder medications. These medications often give the desired pain-relief, but may also cause drowsiness, nausea, vomiting, and constipation. Narcotics may lead to physical and emotional dependence and should be used for limited times only under close supervision.

For those who do not like the expense, the side effects, or the over-dependence on pills, what other ways are there to deal with pain?

One way to cope with pain is to focus on something else. This is something like counting sheep to fall asleep. When my dentist starts drilling, I count to myself, 1, 2, 3, 4, 5 . . . and my attention is taken away from my mouth. Other people prefer saying a prayer, their name, or a favorite word over and over again. Another way to relax and let pain drift away is with visualization, imagining a pleasurable situation or experience. Maybe you would like to be on the beach, lying on the sand, listening to wave after wave hit the shore. Maybe you grew up on a farm and like to remember how peaceful it was at sunrise just before the farm awakened. Would you rather be in the mountains, the woods, or out in a sailboat? What setting is relaxing to you and would help you to feel warm and secure? Picture it. After awhile take a look at your pain and see that it has lost some of its intensity.

Prayer, for some, provides a peaceful experience of concentrating on something other than unpleasant bodily sensations. Among the many other ways of distracting yourself are reading a book, watching TV, knitting, or writing letters. You know what activities you enjoy and find engrossing.

Stress or tension can cause pain or increase pain that is already there. Sometimes there is a vicious circle where you have pain, worry about it, tense up, hurt more and worry more. Breathing techniques can break that cycle. Find a quiet area where you will not be disturbed. Sit up in a comfortable position and lightly place your hands on your belly. Breathe and feel your hand moving out and in. Listen to your breathing, feel it, be lulled by it.

Another technique also begins with your finding a comfortable position and breathing normally a few times. Then take in a very deep breath, hold it to the count of five, and let it all the way out. Now take some slow easy breaths, in your nose and out through your mouth. End with another really deep breath — all the way in, hold it to 5, and out. Breathe in calmness, breathe out tension.

Heart rate, blood pressure, blood flow to the brain, and degree of pain felt all change for the better when you relax. With the technique known as biofeedback, you can "see your relaxation" on a machine. For example, a thermometer attached to your finger will register a higher temperature when you relax. By finding a way to "make the thermometer hotter," you improve your circulation, relieve your headache, relax your whole body. Other devices can help teach you how to lower your blood pressure or feel less pain.

A centuries-old Chinese method of pain-relief, acupuncture, is currently being met with great interest and acceptance in the West. It involves the use of delicate needles inserted into the body to stimulate certain energy pathways or meridians, and block the sensation of pain. A variation of this healing approach, acupressure, is performed by pressing firmly with the fingertips along the same meridians.

What can be done about the plain old headache? Start with the fresh air test. Go outside or to an open window and take a few deep breaths. Sometimes a headache is caused by carbon monoxide, a faulty heating system, a crowded smoke-filled room, or a tension-creating gathering. With fresh air and a change of scenery the headache is relieved.

When you are upset, you tighten your shoulder, neck and head muscles, interfering with blood circulation to the brain and often causing headaches. A massage of shoulders, neck, temples, scalp, and forehead, as described in Chapter 22, helps to loosen those muscles. A warm bath may also be helpful. Some headaches are caused by low blood sugar, by hunger. The remedy for them? Sit down and eat something.

Heavy consumption of caffeine may cause headaches, as well as cause irritability, intestinal disturbances and irregular heartbeats. Juices, decaffeinated coffee, and chamomile tea are good alternatives to coffee.

If any headache lasts a long time or comes back frequently, check with your physician. The pain might be the first clue that you have high blood pressure, sinus problems, allergies, or a vision problem.

Another common area for pain is the back. Being overweight causes extra strain on the spine and can lead to backaches. So can poor posture. Swimming, yoga, and the exercises described in Chapter 1 are excellent ways to relieve pain, to strengthen the back, and to relax.

SAFETY CHECK LIST

by Robert Skeist, R. N.

Falls, motor vehicle accidents, fires and other accidents lead to the deaths each year of more than 25,000 people in our country over the age of 65, as many as die from diabetes and pneumonia. "The time needed for healing and return of function," explains safety expert Dr. Manuel Rodstein, "are greatly prolonged in the aged and the number and severity of complications, such as infection, heart failure, pneumonia and disorientation increased."

Here is a checklist of ways to improve safety in your home and in the homes of your friends and family.

To Prevent Falls:

- Tack carpets down.
- Remove throw rugs or use no-skid backing.
- Remove books, bottles, and other items from the floor.
- Arrange furniture to leave clear paths for walking.
- Install grab-bars by bathtubs and toilets.

- Tack down all stair coverings.
- Have plenty of light in stairways.
- Paint outside steps with a mixture of sand and paint for better traction.
- Avoid loose-fitting trailing robes and poor-fitting shoes and slippers.
- When you get up out of bed, first sit on the side of the bed and dangle your feet. If you are dizzy or light-headed, steady yourself with your hands and wait until your head clears. Then put both feet on the floor and stand up slowly. Check your balance; then start walking.
- Report any dizziness to your doctor, and ask him or her to check all your medications.

To Prevent Motor Vehicle Accidents When You Are Walking:

- Wait for a new green light to cross the street.
- Cross the street only at corners.
- Be especially careful in the evening; most pedestrians are hurt between 6 and 9 p.m. Buy reflective stripping made for construction workers and tape it around the arms of your coats.
- When there is snow and ice on the roads, do not step out into the street until you see the cars not just slow down, but actually stop.

To Prevent Motor Vehicle Accidents When You Are Driving:

- As much as possible, drive when it is light out. (Night vision decreases with aging.)
- Avoid playing the radio or having your windows completely closed so you can hear cars and people better. (Hearing decreases with aging.)
- Allow a greater distance to slow down and stop.
- Stick with roads or highway lanes where you are comfortable with the driving speed.
- Consider taking the "Driver Improvement Program" of the American Association for Retired Persons, which provides four two-hour classes for only $4.00.

To Prevent Fires:

- Never smoke when you are sleepy.
- Keep storage areas clear of rubbish. Store oily rags in covered metal containers.
- Clean lint from the clothes dryer.
- Place portable room heaters away from curtains.
- Repair or replace damaged electrical cords.

For further information, contact:
> National Safety Council
> 440 North Michigan Avenue
> Chicago, Illinois 60611

For information on driving lessons, contact:
> AARP-NRTA
> Driver Improvement Program
> 1225 Connecticut Avenue N. W.
> Suite 401
> Washington, D. C. 20036

SURVIVING VACATIONS, SUMMER'S HEAT AND WINTER'S CHILL

by Robert Skeist, R. N.

It is an old joke that by the time you get back from a vacation, you need another one to recuperate. Here are some guidelines for having a healthy trip and coming home in one piece, followed by summer and winter health advice.

Aloha, doctor. See your general physician and discuss where you will be going, how much you plan to exert yourself, and how long you expect to be gone.

If you have not seen the dentist during the past six months, do so now, so that the pleasure of your trip is not interrupted by a toothache or by poor-fitting dentures.

An infectious idea. If you will be traveling abroad, call your board of health to find out what inoculations you will need. Get your shots at least a month in advance, in case you need time to recover from a bad reaction.

Your health department will provide you with a vaccination certification booklet. Have your doctor fill it in and sign it, then have it authorized by the health department.

No, I am not a drug pusher! Carrying your prescription drugs in an unlabeled pillbox may lead a customs official or a policeman to suspect you of dope-smuggling. To be safe — with your health, as well as with these officials — carry each of your medications in a separate, properly-labeled, unbreakable bottle.

Sometimes a trip is unexpectedly extended, so take along more medication than you think you will need. If you run out of pills, or if your medicines are lost, your "insurance" will be your prescriptions. Ask your doctor for a typed prescription, with generic name and metric dosage, for each of your medicines.

Your medicines will be safer in your purse or carry-on bag, rather than in an airplane luggage compartment (too cold) or a bus luggage compartment (perhaps too hot). Digitalis, insulin, and other emergency medications should be very easy to get to.

Diarrhea and vomiting. Now that I have your attention, I suggest that you ask your doctor for a supply of medications to treat "the runs" (especially if you will be traveling out of the country or to a region where the diet is unfamiliar) and "motion sickness" (especially if you will be flying or traveling on a boat for the first time).

Harold's not drunk, he's a diabetic! Let a friend

know of your health conditions. Carry a card in your wallet listing all of your conditions and medications, as described in Chapter 26. A bracelet indicating your health condition is another safety precaution.

That's not a cow, it's a Civil War cannon! If you sit on your glasses or drop a contact lens and can not tell the Grand Canyon from Lake Michigan, a spare pair or a clearly written prescription can save the day.

I need a doctor! To find an English-speaking doctor abroad, call the United States, Canadian, or British consulate. Get the doctor's full name, address, and receipts for bills. For extra security, you may want to locate a doctor as soon as you arrive in a new area.

When your feet ache, you ache all over. Nothing can wreck a trip like a foot full of blisters. Bring along cotton socks and comfortable walking shoes. If you need a new pair, buy jogging shoes or low-heeled leather shoes, and break them in a month before you travel. Take walks each day, building up gradually from 15 minutes to a total of two hours, so you do not spend your vacation huffing and puffing to keep up with a group.

Don't touch me! On your first few days at the Indiana Dunes, Miami Beach or Waikiki, avoid getting too much sun. Wear a hat, especially if you are bald or have very thin hair. When buying suntan lotion, follow the guidelines described later in this chapter to choose a lotion that shields you from burning sun rays. If you do get burned, get extra rest and drink plenty of liquids. Have a friend apply cool moist towels, then pat dry, spread on Vitamin E cream, and protect your skin from the sun.

So this is Montezuma's revenge. Diarrhea and other digestive troubles are a common reaction to eating bacteria we are not used to in other parts of the world. In Central and South America, Asia, Africa, and when in doubt, avoid raw meats, milk, ice cream, cream sauces, soft cheese, tap water, ice cubes, leafy vegetables, and peeled fruits. Bottled water, beer, boiled water (as in coffee and tea), fruit that you peel yourself, and cooked meats are safer. Go easy on the alcohol and coffee, since they can tire you out.

For diabetics, here are a few special suggestions:

"Soy diabetico." If you are traveling outside of the U.S., learn at least these phrases in the native language: "I am a diabetic." "Sugar or orange juice, please." "Please get me to a doctor."

"No, that's not lemonade." Bring supplies for urine testing and materials needed to test blood from a finger prick.

"Ouch!" Good foot care is extremely important. At a local park or on the sands of Southern California, protect your feet with sandals when the sand

is hot or where there are sharp pebbles or seashells.

Avoid new shoes or overwalking. If you develop a blister, do not pop it. Cover it with gauze and a band-aid, wear loose shoes, and do a minimum of walking for a day or two. Soak your feet in warm water three times a day.

"No, not for heroin!" If you take insulin, take along a letter from your doctor explaining that you are a diabetic and need syringes. This note will come in handy if you go through customs, are stopped by police, or must buy additional syringes in a pharmacy.

"It's four o'clock here, but in Chicago it's two." If you fly through several time zone changes, you may need to adjust your insulin doses. Here is one good method: Keep your watch set according to the time of your departure site. When you arrive at your destination, if more than 24 hours have passed since your last dose, take a few extra units of regular insulin. Then set your watch to the new time zone and take insulin at your normal times. If less than 24 hours have passed since your last dose, then after arrival set your watch to the new time zone and take a little less insulin than usual. Then return to your normal routine.

Check with your doctor for further advice, and listen to the messages your body sends to your mind concerning the temporary need for more insulin or more food. If you need food on a plane when it is not their regular mealtime, tell the stewardess you are a diabetic and must have food now.

No, you can't have my extra orange! Always have carbohydrates with you, such as oranges, graham crackers, hard candy, fruit juice, or sugar cubes.

Time for another taco! As at home, adjust your insulin dosage according to your level of activity, amount of eating, and time of eating. If you don't understand the importance of the "how-to's" of the food-exercise-insulin balance, learn before you travel.

Last but not least, some guidelines for travel by the handicapped.

Ask about special services. Many bus, train, airplane, and car rental agencies make special efforts to meet the needs of handicapped people. But you should call in advance, describe your disability, and make reservations and requests for wheelchairs or other equipment. The same advice goes for hotel reservations. In some cases, a doctor's letter is required to prove that it is safe for you to travel on a plane. Whenever possible, leave from and arrive at busy bus, train, or plane terminals during their off-hours.

Leave the driving to them. Both Trailways and Greyhound will let a handicapped traveler and his or her companion travel for one fare, but you must have doctor's letter explaining your need for assistance.

These bus lines also allow for Seeing Eye dogs for blind passengers and Hearing Ear dogs for the deaf.

Drive it yourself. Avis, Hertz, and National all have cars with left and right hand controls, usually without an extra charge. Special cars are limited as services are not available in all parts of the country, so call in advance.

Or travel by rail or air. Many airlines have wheelchairs available and welcome Seeing Eye dogs or Hearing Ear dogs. Amtrak has some train cars equipped for wheelchair entrance.

Additional travel resources for the general public, diabetics, and the handicapped are listed at the end of this chapter.

Summer Health

With or without traveling, summer offers certain pleasures and presents various health risks. I (in my 30's), my parents (in their 60's), and my grandmother (in her 90's) all like to be outside a lot. Walking, swimming, and lying in the sun seem to be membership requirements for being in my family. The same goes for large numbers of older people who head for the sun in Florida or California, in a park or by a lake, to splash in water with grandchildren or relax with a good book.

A certain amount of sunlight is necessary for good health. With a little time outside each day, your body soaks in ultraviolet rays from the sun and produces Vitamin D. This vitamin is used to bring calcium into your teeth and bones. Roasting in the sunlight hour after hour in your lounge chair, however, raises a couple of health and cosmetic issues. It may age your skin, making it drier, thinner, and more wrinkly. Year-after-year exposure to lots of sun may lead to wart-like growths or skin cancer. A more immediate risk is sunburn. As the sun's ultraviolet rays react with your skin's melanin, a tan develops. Overexposure to these same rays causes a burn.

In general, fair-haired, light-skinned, blue-eyed people are most likely to burn (as well as most likely to develop skin cancer). Olive-skinned and even dark brown-skinned people may also burn if they are in the sunlight too often or for long periods.

For those of you who really enjoy the feeling of lying in the sun or the look of a nice tan, I recommend the "easy-does-it" approach. The first time you're out in the sun, limit yourself to 15 minutes at midday (between 10:00 A. M. and 2:00 P. M., when the sun's rays are strongest) or 30 minutes earlier or later in the day. For the next several days, as long as you're not burning at all, you can increase the time by 15 minutes.

Protect your skin with a *sunscreen*. Baby oil, mineral oil, and hand lotion are fine to use to moisten your skin when you are back inside, but they do not protect you from the sun's ultraviolet rays. Nor do most suntan lotions protect you from burning. To select the right product for you, check the package for the Sun Protection Factor (SPF). (See chart below.) Sunscreen or suntan lotion should be applied each one to two hours in the sun, and after sweating or swimming. Delicate-skinned people or those with any allergies should test any new lotion by rubbing it onto a small area of their body and letting it stay overnight. If the area is then red or tender, try a different product.

Tan, Don't Burn

Select a lotion that is labeled with the Sun Protection Factor (SPF) you need. This chart is based on information provided by the U. S. Food and Drug Administration (FDA).

If you...	Choose a Lotion with SPF number
Always burn easily and never tan	15 or more
Always burn easily and barely tan	8-14
Burn easily and get a light tan	6-7
Tan gradually and burn moderately	4-5
Always tan well and burn minimally	3
Tan dark brown and rarely burn	2

"In practical terms," states the FDA, "a person who usually gets red after 20 minutes should be able to stay in the sun for two hours if he or she applies a sunscreen with a rating of '6,' provided the product is not washed or sweated off. A product with a rating of '4' will permit a person to stay in the sun without getting a sunburn four times longer than without a sunscreen. Once a person's skin has become accustomed to the sun, a product with less protective capacity may be used."

Some people are attracted to products containing DHA (dihydroxyacetone) that boast of the ability to tan you indoors. I suggest you stay away from these. The "tan" they give may be yellow, orange, or blotchy, and it will not protect you from burning.

If you do, in spite of this advice, get sunburned, your skin will feel warm and sore, and you may be hit with fever, chills, nausea, and fatigue. For a simple home treatment, drink plenty of water and get some extra rest. Have a friend soak towels in cool water, wring them out, and lay them on your burned areas. A cool washcloth on your forehead will also feel good. After 10 or 15 minutes, remove the towels and let your skin dry by exposure to the air. Aspirin or acetaminophen (available as a generic or by brand names including Tylenol and Datril) may also be used to bring down a fever and relieve pain.

A little vinegar dabbed onto the skin is an old home remedy to take the sting out. Non-scented lotions and oils may be used to restore moisture to your skin. Vitamin E cream rubbed gently into the burned skin twice a day for two days will help the skin heal quickly.

A special warning about sunburn should be given to anyone taking medications with the side effect called *photosensitivity*. Examples of such drugs are chlorpromazine (Thorazine), hydrochlorothiazide (Esidrex, Hydrodiuril, Oretic), tetracycline, erythromycin, the sulfas, barbiturates, quinine, quinidine, psoralens, demeclocycline, and promethazine. Sunlight striking the skin of someone taking any of these medications may cause a severe burn. Discuss this issue with your pharmacist and your physician. It may be necessary to avoid sunbathing, use an effective sunscreen lotion, and wear a hat and protective clothing when outdoors.

If you look forward to more exercise in the summer, great! So do I. It is a fine time to walk or bicycle around your neighborhood, through the parks, or along the lakeshore. But the hotter it is outside — especially if it is very humid — the more strenuous it is to exercise. Lightweight and light-colored clothing will keep you more comfortable. To keep the sun from beating directly on your head — especially important for those who are bald or have thinning hair — a summer hat helps a lot. And plan your walk or other exercise for when it is cooler, before 10:00 A. M. or after 2:00 P. M.

A lot of people believe that it is harmful to drink water before and during exercise. In fact, the opposite is true. The Chicago Heart Association recommends that you "drink water freely both before exercise and every 15-30 minutes or when moderate thirst occurs."

At times, exercising under the hot sun may leave you feeling dizzy, faint, off-balance, nauseous, exhausted, confused, or upset, or you may have muscle cramps. These may be signs that you have lost too much water and body heat. At this point (and hopefully well before this point), the thing to do is get shade, water, and rest. If the symptoms do not go away after half an hour, call your doctor.

If you are taking a diuretic (commonly known as a "water pill" and often used to treat high blood pressure), pay special attention to summer exercise precautions. Ask your doctor to check your blood chemistry; for some people, summer sweating calls for a change in diuretic dosage.

Air pollution, especially from ozone, is a summer health issue for people living in areas with lots of industry or traffic. Ozone is a colorless, stinky, poisonous gas released into the air in dangerous amounts by automobiles and industry. It irritates the air passages in the lungs, making it harder to breathe, easier to get infections, and making asthma attacks and heart attacks more likely.

Ozone hits hardest on hot humid days between 11:00 A. M. and 6:00 P. M.

To reduce the impact of this pollution on your health, you can do your walking in mid-morning or after the evening rush hour, and stop smoking. If you have chest pain, shortness of breath, or extreme fatigue, go to bed and call your doctor.

I really should not have to give this advice. The burden should not be on the individual to cope with poisoned air. We must join together to fight for stricter industrial pollution guidelines, better emission controls on automobiles, and a drastic cutback in automobile traffic together with improved public transportation, to make breathing safe for everyone.

If you are concerned about body odor, your best bet is daily washing with ordinary soap and water. Many of the soaps sold as special "antiperspirant" or "antiseptic" products have been shown to cause side effects including skin irritations and greater likelihood for sunburn. According to Consumers Union, $40,000,000 per year is spent to advertise antiperspirants, many of which are useless or even harmful. Again, stick to plain soap and water.

Next on the list of possible summer aggravations is heat rash, with itchy, burning skin, fever, and fatigue. To avoid it, wear loose-fitting clothes made of natural fibers — cotton "breathes" much better than polyester. Underwear and socks, especially, should be cotton and changed at least once a day. The summer calls for showering more frequently. Cornstarch dusted lightly on particularly sweaty areas of your body will help absorb the moisture.

If you do develop a heat rash, be sure to get some extra rest. Bathe often in cool water, pat yourself dry, and lie naked exposed to the air on clean sheets.

When it comes to food, it is natural and healthy to eat more lightly in the summertime. Grains, beans, cold soups, and lots of salad "set well." Try barbecuing fish instead of hamburger, drinking fruit juice or iced herbal tea instead of soda pop, and eating fresh fruits for dessert.

Winter Health

As I complete this chapter, eight inches of snow have just fallen on Chicago. The air is calm, but strong winds are predicted for later this week. It is time for some practical suggestions to help readers avoid winter colds, shortness of breath, and heart strain.

Eat well. Be sure to have some foods every day that are rich in Vitamin C, such as oranges, grapefruit, tangerines, broccoli, and green peppers. When you come in from the cold, do not reach for coffee and doughnuts, since sugar and caffeine give you energy for a little while, then leave you tired and depressed. Instead, try toast and peanut butter with juice or a piece of fruit. At mealtimes, fix foods like grains, beans, fish, chicken, hearty soups, stew, and vegetables. When you have plans to go outside, have a good meal about 1 1/2 hours before leaving home.

Keep your home warm. Insulation around the windows and doors is very important to prevent drafts. Drapes help, too, as do carpets on the floor. If you use space heaters or your oven for heat, have them checked for safety, and be sure you have ventilation for gases.

Humidify. Heat from central heating, space heater, and radiators dries the air. This causes drying of the mucus membranes of your nose, mouth, and throat. Next may come coughing, sore throats, and the formation of mucus plugs that clog tiny air passageways in your lungs and make breathing more difficult. Preventing these problems is especially important for people with chronic respiratory diseases.

A small humidifier can be purchased for as little as $10.00 to $15.00 (less if you can find one second-hand or on sale). Keep it in your bedroom at night, then in whatever room you use most during the day. Clean it often, and follow directions to prevent the build-up of molds and fungi.

You can humidify at almost no expense by placing a foil roasting pan or any old baking dish on top of a space heater or radiator and keeping it filled with water. In your kitchen, a large water-filled soup pot over a very low flame will help. Another effective humidifier can be made in five minutes with a bucket, an old newspaper, scissors, and string. Roll up the paper, tie a string around its middle, and stand it upright in the bucket. Make several six-inch cuts starting at the top of the paper, so it opens like a flower. When you fill the bucket with water, it will travel up the newspaper and evaporate into the air.

Protect your heart and lungs when you go outside. If you have a respiratory problem, breathing in very cold air through your mouth may shock the warm bronchi (breathing passages) and cause spasms, shortness of breath, and coughing. Make a point of breathing through your nose, so the air is warmed and humidified when it reaches your lungs. An air-warming mask or a scarf over your mouth are other ways to protect your lungs.

If you have any heart or lung problem, walk more slowly than usual and carry groceries or other items in a shopping cart. Dress in layers: shirt, sweater, and coat on top, long underwear and pants on bottom. Forget about any notion of "fashion" that prevents you from wearing warm sensible clothes that fully cover your legs. Be sure also to wear a hat or scarf, so you do not lose your body's heat through a bare head. Rubber boots are good to keep your feet warm and dry and to give you extra traction on icy sidewalks.

Walk safely. With aging may come poor eyesight,

reduced strength and coordination, and worsened hearing. Many people, particularly women after the menopause, also develop more brittle bones due to osteoporosis, which slows down the healing process after accidents. Winter in the North brings snow and ice, slippery sidewalks, and dangerous driving conditions. There are, though, several ways to make your walk a safer one.

Stairs and sidewalks should be kept clear. If you live in a building where services are supposed to be provided by a landlord, ask that snow be shoveled each day it falls. If necessary, have several people in the building call the landlord until the walks are clean. Ask that a bag of salt or sand be kept in the hallway so you can scoop it out when necessary onto slippery steps.

I recommend rubbers or boots with rough soles. Smooth-soled shoes, and shoes or boots with more than one-inch heels, make it easier to fall. On your way outside, stop in the doorway and look at how icy the stairs and sidewalks are. Use handrails if they are provided, and go slowly until you get a good feel for the walking conditions. At night or on slippery patches, take small steps. If you do fall when you are out walking, do your best to relax your body and roll on your side as you hit the ground.

Not only is snow hard on walkers, it presents serious problems for drivers. It is harder to see other cars or people crossing in front of you and takes much longer to stop. If a car coming toward you has a stop sign, wait until you see that the car actually stops intead of skidding into the intersection. Most pedestrian accidents occur at dusk or night. Wearing a light-colored coat with refletive tape around your arms or legs will make it easier for drivers to see you.

Stay in touch with friends. Love, touch, and companionship are basic human needs at all stages in life. Friendly contact with people not only makes you feel better, it builds up your resistance against colds. Take two kisses and call me in the morning.

For more information, write or call:

Senior Travel Tips
Discovery Travel
120 East Ogden Avenue
Hinsdale, Illinois 60521
(Chicago phone: (312) 242-1847)
(Suburban phone: (312) 920-9730)

How to Fly
Air Transport Association of America
1709 New York Avenue, N. W.
Washington, D. C. 20006
(General information on air travel, with section entitled "Health and Age No Barrier to Air Travel.")

Medication Safety Card
Seniors' Health Program
Augustana Hospital
411 West Dickens Avenue
Chicago, Illinois 60614

Medic Alert Foundation International
Turlock, California 95380
Phone: (209) 632-2371

For information on the Medic Alert bracelet or necklace system for identifying health information useful in an emergency.

Travelers Aid Association of America
44 East 23rd Street
New York, N. Y. 10010
(Provides counseling, information, and direction services to people in trouble away from home.)

IAMAT (International Association for Medical
   Assistance to Travelers)
Empire State Building
350 Fifth Avenue — Suite 5620
New York, N. Y. 10001
American Diabetes Association
600 Fifth Avenue
New York, N. Y. 10020
(for "Travel Tips for Diabetics," a pamphlet.)

A variety of special information for handicapped travelers is available:

Travel Tips for the Handicapped
United States Travel Service
U. S. Department of Commerce
Washington, D. C. 20230

Access Amtrak
Amtrak Public Affairs
955 L'Enfant Plaza, S. W.
Washington, D. C. 20024
(Call toll-free: (800) 523-5720)

Helping Hand
Director of Customer Relations
Greyhound Lines
Greyhound Tower
Phoenix, Arizona 85077
Phone: (602) 248-2920

Good Samaritan
Continental Trailways
1512 Commerce Street
Dallas, Texas 75201
Phone: (214) 655-7900

Avis Rent-A-Car
(Call toll-free: (800) 331-1212)

Hertz Rent-A-Car
(Call toll-free: (800) 654-3131)

National Rent-A-Car
(Call toll-free: (800) 328-4567)

Air Travel for the Handicapped
TransWorld Airlines
1100 Connecticut Avenue, N. W.
Washington, D. C. 20036
(Information for travel on TWA, but much of it applies to other airlines.)

*Access Travel: A Guide to Accessibility of Airport
  Terminals*
Architectural Transportation Barriers
  Compliance Board
Washington, D. C. 20201
(A directory of airports with facilities for handicapped and elderly. Information is updated quarterly and published in "Travel Planner and Hotel/Motel Guide," a Reuben H. Donnelley publication received by many travel agents.)

A List of Guidebooks for Handicapped Travelers
President's Committee on Employment of the
  Handicapped
1111 20th and L Streets, N. W.
Vanguard Building
Washington, D. C. 20210

Access National Parks
Superintendent of Documents
U. S. Government Printing Office
Washington, D. C. 20402
(Covers more than 300 parks, battlefields, and monuments.)

Society for the Advancement of Travel for the
  Handicapped
26 Court Street
Brooklyn, New York 11242
Phone: (212) 858-5483
(Updated listings of city directories and companies which have tours for disabled travelers.)

FEELINGS

CHANGES IN WOMEN'S LIVES: ROSE'S STORY

by Ruth Huang, R. N.

I have shared many special moments with my friend Rose Myria. During the blue days of my pregnancy, she was a constant source of comfort with her phone calls and visits. At my son's home birth, she arrived with a bag of gifts: a dozen red roses, a space heater (it was the Blizzard of '79 in Chicago!), ice chips, massage oil, a bath robe, records, and a camera. She answered the telephone, informing friends of the progress of my labor, as she baked her first challah, a loaf of bread for the baby's first blessing. After the delivery, she sat and massaged my feet. She also took one of my son's first photos — Samuel, one half-hour old, being held in a tub of warm water and stretching his legs for the first time. Sharing my birth experience was especially meaningful to Rose. She had had four natural childbirths and breastfed her infants, and now wanted to give me support.

But this is Rose! She is a nurturing and energetic person. This is one of the reasons she has been highly successful in her practice as an Esalen-style masseuse. She is sensitive to the needs of others. She transmits this sensitivity through her hands with a gentle, non-threatening, and healing touch. "Trust your touch" is her motto, and trusting her touch has given her a unique career and lifestyle for the past eight years.

"Sometimes I wonder what my life would have been like . . . ," Rose mused in her kitchen over a cup of tea and conversation about the changes in her life. We both laughed.

Eight years ago, Rose was "just Rosie." She was the wife of a successful businessman and the mother of four grown children. She had spent her adult life raising children, caring for her husband and household, and doing volunteer work. Then one day, after an evening at the movies, her husband asked for a divorce.

"It was a complete surprise," Rose told me. "I knew we were growing apart, but the signs did not seem relevant to the total structure of our life. I was typically confused and hurt, yet supportive of him. I thought he was going through male menopause or problems with business. I sought out reasons why. In the beginning I was not considering giving him a divorce. I was anticipating a redefinition of our relationship. I was seeking answers from him. Later, when I realized our relationship was over, I was suddenly very angry. There hadn't been any talking. It was his decision for our marriage to end."

Rosie was 45 years old then. Her marriage of 22 years was over. Her children were away at school. She was alone in her house.

Rose's first year on her own was filled with tears and confusion, with questioning and exploring. She had to fill her time, face the rest of her life, and find a way to earn money. She joined a women's rap group, took part in human potential workshops, and decided to give dancing a try. Off she went to classes in belly dancing, jazz, and hula. "I was always the oldest one in the class," Rose said. "It didn't seem to bother the other women — mostly in their twenties — and it didn't bother me. In all of these dance classes, I learned to stretch and to enjoy moving around. Four years before my divorce, both of my shoulders ached from bursitis, but dancing seemed to cure it. It also toned my belly, which is the first place to go with a lot of women . . . and men!

"Dancing put me in touch with my body," Rose continued. "From there I got interested in massage." She took a few massage classes, volunteered her time at the Jewish Community Center, got a part-time job at a health club, and launched a career. She had always enjoyed being creative. She had studied art in college. She had raised four children, "and what could be more creative or important than that?" She found she enjoyed "touching and giving form to a person's body" through massage.

Through ads in a women's newspaper, Rose found new clients. She wrote articles for a local paper. She slowly expanded her practice to include massage and sensory awareness workshops for women, couples, and nurses.

Other aspects of life have also become important to Rose in the eight years since her divorce. She has rediscovered herself as an attractive woman and as a woman who can once again have relationships with men. She has developed close women friends and a network of friends who do massage, therapy, and body work. She has also learned to find pleasure in her time alone. Rose Myria, her chosen professional name, identifies this new woman.

Looking ahead, Rose is excited and busy making plans. There are different types of massage and body work to study and more writing she is interested in doing. She has ideas for developing her massage practice and workshops. Her evolving relationships are enjoyable. Rose laughs. She is 53 years old, facing new challenges, and enjoying her life!

The mid-40's through the mid-60's are challenging — if not depressing or bewildering — for most women. This is the time of the climacteric or "change of life," a period in the life cycle that presents women with many experiences that may threaten their sense of identity and self-esteem.

The physical changes women face are dramatic. Female hormones, the estrogens and progesterones that control a woman's menstrual cycle, decline. These hormones are involved with the feminine, youthful appearance of the body, the soft, firm skin, feminine curves and the development of the sexual organs. With the decrease in female hormones, menstruation, — over a period of years or of months — stops, and one faces the fact that the potential for child bearing is over. The hormonal changes may lead to a thinning and drying of the lining of the vagina. A loss of calcium from the bones is also possible, leading to more brittle bones and an increased risk of broken hips.

About half of all menopausal women experience hot flashes or flushes, sudden changes in body temperature. For each woman the experience is different. It may be a warm glow or intense heat with perspiration, last moments or several minutes, occur once in a while or several times a day.

For many years a medication response to menopause known as ERT — Estrogen Replacement Therapy — has been popular, especially among middle class and wealthier women. They have hoped to preserve youthful appearance and to avoid some of the physical changes associated with menopause. In recent years, though, these drugs have been strongly linked to an increased risk of cancer of the uterus. In addition, there is no proof that ERT does in fact keep women young.

Dr. J. Richard Crout, Director of the U. S. Food and Drug Administration's Bureau of Drugs, suggests that a woman "should discuss with her physician whether she needs to take or remain on estrogen. There are some valid uses for estrogen," he maintains. "Treatment of menopausal symptons — particularly 'hot flashes' — for a period of months is clearly a common and acceptable practice. But beyond that a woman is taking a risk of cancer for a false promise of maintaining youthfulness."

I asked Rose how this information related to her own experience with menopause. Her periods stopped two years ago, she told me. She did not experience hot flashes, headaches, or any unpleasant physical sensations. She has not taken any medications in relation to menopause. Her dancing has helped keep her bones strong and her muscles toned.

But what about her emotions? Even though most women at age 45 or 55 have no desire to have more children, it comes as a shock to some that the choice is no longer theirs. This may be experienced as a loss of femininity. It may also be experienced as a reminder of aging, "which most of us are aware of and have mixed feelings about from the time we turn 30," Rose said. Yet she also found a positive side to menopause: "I'm free of the minor inconvenience of my period, and what's the greatest is that

I can enjoy sex without birth control and not have the slightest concern about getting pregnant."

Today, many thousands of women are faced with their own menopause and aging, the challenge of developing their own identities, the responsibility of writing their own stories. This is Rose's story, one of rebirth.

To hear from the "new voice for middle years and older women," a group active against ageism and sexism and working for dramatic improvements in the health and economic situation of women, contact:

> Tish Sommers
> Older Women's League Educational Fund
> 3800 Harrison Street
> Oakland, California 94611.

We especially recommend their "GRAY PAPER No. 3 — Older Women and Health Care: Issues for Survival."

For additional readings on menopause, see:

> *Our Bodies, Ourselves* by the Boston Women's Health Collective, Simon and Schuster, New York, N. Y., $2.95.

Also recommended as a very clear book is:

> *A Clinical Guide to the Menopause and Post Menopause*, Agenst Laboratories Information Publishing Company, New York, N. Y.

Literature on related topics is available from

National Action Forum for Older Women
c/o Nancy King
1120 Francis Scott Key Hall
University of Maryland
College Park, Maryland 20742

SEX AT ANY AGE

by Barbara Giovannoni, and
Joseph Giovannoni, R. N.

"Goodnight, Mom! Goodnight, Walter!"

"Goodnight kids. Drive carefully."

Janice turned to Bill as they got into their car. "Did you see the way Walter was touching Mom?"

"Yeah, he stroked her arm so tenderly, so sensuously," Bill answered, starting the car and pulling out of the driveway. "And every time your mother spoke to Walter they looked almost romantic."

Janice thought about her mother and this new man in her life. "You know, Bill, I thought Mom was too old for that kind of stuff. Dad died seven years ago. She's almost 70, and Walter is 73! It's cute when they cuddle, but I got the feeling they're going to spend the night together!"

They came to a stoplight, Bill lit up a cigarette and turned to his wife. "I had that same feeling," he said, "but it's real hard for me to believe that old folks like that would be interested in anything more than holding hands."

Many people, regardless of age, share the attitude of Janice and Bill. They think that sex automatically ends at some magical age like 60, or with the death of a spouse. Some believe that older people do not or should not desire sex. They may call sexually active old people "showoffs" or dismiss them as "cute." These attitudes harm us all, old and young, who need warmth, affection, love and human touch.

During a recent presentation on sexuality before a senior citizens' club, we asked, "When do you want sexual activity to end for you?" Three quarters of the men and women gave answers along the lines of "Never!" and "When I'm dead!" Pfeiffer's 1974 study produced similar results: eight out of ten men in their late 60's continued to be interested in sex, and seven out of ten, married or unmarried, were sexually active. Women in that study who still lived with their husbands also expressed strong sexual interest.

Why are these people still sexual? After all, most women over fifty cannot bear children. And older men, even if they're involved with younger women, are seldom eager to wake up in the middle of the night to feed and walk a crying infant. But sex is not simply for reproduction. It is a wonderful way of communicating and expressing affection. It helps us feel good, alive, desirable, worthy. Dr. Domeena Renshaw of Loyola University's Sexual Dysfunction Clinic adds that "sex is our body's natural tranquilizer." It releases tension and helps relieve frustration, hostility and depression.

Then why have some older people stopped having sex? "Ever since my husband died 25 years ago I'm not interested in any man," a 90-year old woman told us. "I was married. My husband died. That's that." She is not alone in her attitude. Widowhood, Pfeiffer found, is frequently the reason older women stop having sex. But the pain and difficulties of losing her husband need not prevent a woman from finding sexual satisfaction. Remarriage, affairs with older or younger men, loving relationships with women, and masturbation are all options to consider.

Ignorance of the body's functioning is another barrier to sexual pleasure. Men often fear that age automatically brings impotence, and this "performance anxiety" itself may be enough to prevent an erection. In reality, the vast majority of older men can enjoy erections and orgasms. They may take longer, but this can bring added pleasure to the man and his partner. An older woman may notice that her vagina is dry or that it hurts during sexual intercourse and conclude that sex ends with menopause. She may not know about treatments available to improve lubrication of the vagina and may never have learned how to stimulate the clitoris for sexual satisfaction. When this ignorance is swept away, some older people enjoy sex more than ever before.

Fear of physical danger or of the disapproval of others are additional factors that hold some people back. "I don't want to overdo it and get a heart attack," one man states, although many doctors believe that most people who can climb two flights of stairs without huffing and puffing can easily handle the excitement of sex. "And I'm embarrassed to talk about it with my doctor. He might think I'm dirty," the man continues. But his doctor's job includes honestly answering questions from patients. And that the phrase "dirty old man" should go into the same wastebasket as other insults like "kike" or "nigger". We live in a society where youth is "in" and wrinkles are "out." This stops many of us from seeing the beauty of a face, of a body, of a person who has lived several decades.

We sometimes fear most of all the reactions of our own children. Leah Shaefer found that youngsters and even middle-aged people are often uncomfortable with the notion that their parents actually "do that!" This is especially true in those families where the parents were uncomfortable talking about sex or touching each other fondly in front of their kids. A child may be nervous about an older parent's sexuality because of his or her own fears of aging, boredom with sex, unresolved grief over the loss of one parent, or even out of fear that the widowed parent's lover may inherit the family savings.

Finally, some older people, as Pfeiffer found, stop sexual activity simply because they don't enjoy it. "I never liked sex much and I simply don't want it now," a 67-year old woman told us. Sex should stop "the sooner the better," agreed one man we spoke with. Another woman recently asked us, "Why do some young people try to push sex on us? OK, so now it's 'in' to be 'liberated', but I'm not interested! Next thing you know you'll be having me keep track of how many orgasms I'm having. I resent the pressure!" These people should not be pressured into sex. They, and each of us, should have a choice. The information in this chapter, drawn from our experiences in nursing, sex counselling, and our own marriage, may help you choose the role sex will play in your life.

Sexual Anatomy

It is not unusual to hear that a woman has never looked at her external sex organs (vulva) or that a man has some misconceptions about his penis. "Know your body," therefore, is the theme of this section.

The vulva is a general term referring to the external female sex organs. The labia majora are the two visible rounded folds or "lips." The outer surface is covered with pubic hair, and the inner surface is smooth and moist. The labia minora are the two

189

inner folds of skin extending around the opening of the vagina and joined at the top to the clitoris. The mons pubis is the raised bony area covered by pubic hair. The urethra — the passageway for urine from the bladder — is located just above the opening of the vagina. The pea-shaped clitoris lies above the urethra at the top of the labia minora. It may be partially covered by the clitoral hood, which can easily be pulled back. The clitoris, with an extensive supply of nerves and blood vessels, can easily become erect.

Research by Masters and Johnson has demonstrated that a woman's orgasm results from direct or indirect stimulation of the clitoris with fingers, a tongue or the movements of sexual intercourse. The vagina has far fewer nerve endings than the clitoris. Its main purpose is for reproduction, while the clitoris has no function other than providing a woman with erotic pleasure.

Many women have never experienced an orgasm because they have never touched, explored and stimulated their sexual organs. Women who seek professional help to achieve orgasm are helped to accept their bodies and to excite themselves by masturbating. They learn to know their anatomy, to find out what pleases them sexually, and to communicate openly with their partners.

The penis and scrotum are the man's external sex organs. The scrotum is a pouch containing the testicles, which produce sperm and the male hormone, testosterone.

The sperm travel upward through two tubes called the vas deferens. They come together below the bladder, where they join the seminal vesicle and then the tube from the bladder that carries urine. The prostate gland surrounds the junction of these tubes. In the prostate, fluids from the seminal vesicles and the prostate mix with sperm to form the thick whitish fluid called semen. The prostate squeezes semen into the urethra during an orgasm.

Some men are very concerned about penis size. Often, penises that are different sizes shen relaxed are about the same size during erections. Regardless of size, the penis can be contained in a vagina without a feeling of empty space, since the vaginal walls touch each other.

The uncircumcised penis has a foreskin which can be pulled over the head of the penis. During erections the foreskin tightens and pulls back. To prevent the build-up of a whitish, curdy, foul smelling substance called smegma, an uncircumcised man should pull back his foreskin and clean the area while bathing.

How Aging Affects Sex for Men

The great majority of men can continue enjoying sex into their seventies, eighties, and beyond. In fact, the main causes of male sexual problems — other than diseases, which we will discuss later — are being anxious about sex or having sex too rarely.

A man who expects impotence may become like a spectator of love-making, nervously waiting to see if he can "do it". This naturally makes sex less enjoyable, and may lead a man to avoid or abandon it.

But doesn't sexual functioning change as a man grows older? Yes. The basic change is a slowing down of each step of his orgasm. It takes longer for his penis to grow hard, and it may not become quite as large as it used to during erection. He may produce less fluid to lubricate the tip of the penis and less to spurt out during orgasm. More time may be required for intercourse or masturbation before orgasm is reached, and more time before the man can have another erection.

On the positive side, and older man and his partner may enjoy that he can now "last longer." He may, in his maturity, get greater pleasure from pleasing his partner. He may have more appreciation for touching, holding, kissing, and the sensations of intercourse even when it doesn't lead to orgasm. In short, he may find new meaning in the term "making love."

Good diet, regular exercise, a sense of excitement and meaning in life, and regular intercourse or masturbation will reduce the male sexual slowing down process. The form of intercourse or masturbation is a matter of personality and choice for each man. At some point in their lives, nine out of ten men masturbate to the point of orgasm (Kinsey, Pomeroy, Martin). As men reach their sixties, more of them masturbate (Sadock, Kaplan, Freedman, 1976). Whether a man masturbates himself or his partner masturbates him, it provides pleasure, releases tension, and helps him stay in good shape sexually.

There has so far been little understood about the possibility for happiness in gay (homosexual) relationships among older men. A recent film called "Word Is Out" made a fine contribution in this area, showing two men in their sixties with a very fond, loving relationship. As is true for older men who have relationships with women, older gay men are likely to enjoy life and sexuality more as they find value and beauty in their own lives and in the lives of their friends, and as they share open conversation and gentle touch.

How Aging Affects Sex for Women

Women at any age are capable of sexual excitement and orgasm. In fact, some women experience their first orgasms when they are in their sixties or older. Menopause marks the end of a woman's reproductive cycle including her monthly bleeding;

it does not mark the end of sex. Nor does widowhood necessarily mean the end of sex for a woman.

There are frequently some menopausal changes that affect sexual relations. With less production of the female sex hormone estrogen, the walls of the vagina grow thinner and drier. Pressure from a penis or finger might hurt and possibly cause a little bleeding. The vagina may also lose some of its muscle tone or "grip".

Interestingly, these problems are much less likely to develop for a woman who masturbates or has sexual intercourse once or twice a week. Use of K-Y jelly or other lubricants that dissolve in water (*not* petroleum jelly or other oil-based products) can make masturbation or intercourse more comfortable. It is also important for each woman to let her partner know just what kind of stimulation feels good.

Some doctors prescribe estrogen creams, suppositories, or tablets to treat vaginal dryness and sensitivity. However, the use of too much estrogen may lead to fluid retention, weight gain, upset stomach, headache, and vaginal discharge. More seriously, it increases the risk of developing uterine cancer.

Other chapters in this book deal with a woman's grief over losing her husband and with the emotional impact of developing wrinkles and sagging breasts. These changes need not mean the end of sexual satisfaction for women who appreciate themselves and value their day-to-day lives. Relationships with men, closeness with other women, and masturbation are choices some women make. What kind of emotional sharing, holding and touching, or sexual involvements are right for a given woman? That's something for her to work out with people with whom she can be open.

The Effects of Illness on Sexuality

Certain diseases can lead to sexual problems. For this reason, a complete physical examination is done at centers like Loyola University's Sexual Dysfunction Clinic. Once physical problems have been cleared up, the individual's attention can turn to finding and communicating to the partner what feels good.

Most men have had their prostate glands checked by a physician inserting a gloved finger into the rectum. An enlarged prostate, common in men over 60 in our society, squeezes the urethra and makes urination difficult or painful. Continuing to have orgasms from sexual intercourse or masturbation helps to prevent prostate problems.

When a prostate problem develops, the doctor may recommend prostate massage and warm sitz baths, or perhaps surgery. One possible result of prostate surgery is "dry orgasm," meaning that a man can still enjoy sexual climax but does not spurt out any semen.

Following perineal prostatectomy, many men are unable to have erections. This problem is not caused by the two other types of prostate surgery. We advise men to ask their doctors for complete information on each procedure before deciding on surgery.

Another medical/sexual issue for men is the problem of medication side effects. Certain drugs used to lower blood pressure or to "calm the nerves" may lead to impotence. When possible, a man should understand and cope with his emotions without drugs, or ask his doctor to choose a type and dose of medication that will not interfere with his sexual pleasure. Alcohol is another drug that can cause male impotence. Dr. Robert Butler of the National Institute on Aging recommends that an older man drink no more than 1½ oz. of hard liquor, 12 oz. of wine, or 24 oz. of beer per day.

A heart attack can be serious and frightening, but it is not a reason to give up sex. Many physicians believe that after eight to sixteen weeks it is O. K. to resume sexual activity. A common test used is seeing if the person who suffered a heart attack can now climb two flights of stairs without experiencing chest pain or difficulty in breathing. Stress on the heart will be reduced by avoiding sex after a heavy meal, when drunk or exhausted, in extreme temperatures, or in unfamiliar settings. Lying on one's back or side during sex will also reduce strain on the heart.

Diabetes contributes to sexual problems for some people by interfering with the penis or clitoris becoming erect. Not everyone with diabetes develops this problem, and many with the problem can be helped with sex counselling. Keeping the diabetes under control—with diet, exercise, medication and regular checkups allow most diabetics full sexual functioning.

Arthritis, stroke and backache are three conditions that can make a person feel more achy than sensuous. If you have these problems, a firm mattress, plenty of rest, warm baths, and proper exercises will help you relax. Feeling comfortable is an important part of enjoying another person's touch.

For additional reading, see:

Man's Body — An Owner's Manual by the Diagram Group Paddington Press Ltd. New York, N. Y. $6.95 — An easy to read, heavily illustrated guide to male sex organs, sexuality, aging, and other topics.

Our Bodies, Our Selves by the Boston Women's Health Book, Collective, Simon and Schuster, New York, N. Y., $2.95. The best-selling feminist guide to anatomy, sexuality, relationships, menopause, and women in the health care system.

GRAY AND GAY

by Richard Steinman, Ph. D.

In a society where old people are often regarded as outdated inventory and homosexuals made outcasts, what lies in store for aging lesbians and gay men?

Some paint a bleak picture. They point out that few gay people are parents and grandparents, so they can't call on the younger generations for emotional support, money, or help with day-to-day activities. Non-parents do not have the particular sense of immortality that offspring may provide. Even those gay people who do have children may be cut off from them due to their families' hostile or nervous attitudes or to discriminatory court decisions.

In most working situations, being homosexual has been seen as a serious liability. Many gay people have "lost points" for failing to attend office social events with their families or for not responding to heterosexual flirting or advances. Some have been "discovered" and deemed unfit to continue careers in teaching, child care, or other areas. Such pressures have forced some to change jobs more frequently than they would have wished to, thus building up less economic security in the form of salaries and pensions.

Another difficulty stems from the fact that homosexual relationships are not granted the stamp of approval of the legal system or — with a few recent exceptions — the blessing of religious institutions. Nor are they frequently celebrated in the movies or seen as essential to successful political campaigns. Such negative influences, which were even stronger when today's older gays were growing up, make it quite a challenge for their relationships to survive and provide security. In spite of this, love and friendship often prevail.

Having listed these problems, however, only half the story has been told. Those who have not raised children will naturally not be faced with the crisis of what to do when the children leave home. By the time they enter their 40's or 50's, many gay people will have developed considerable inner resources, strong friendships, and ongoing interests. They are not likely to view sex primarily in relation to bearing children, but to value it for intimacy and pleasure at any age.

Moreover, the post-retirement identity crisis faced by many people — men in particular in today's older generations — may not hit gay people quite so severely. They have already had to deal with another major identity crisis, the challenge of maintaining a secret identity in isolation from traditional patterns that society takes for granted.

Retirement may even be met with a special delight. Menningerode and Adelman quote one older gay man who was eager to end his working days: "That's when I no longer had to hide my homosexuality, and I went out and celebrated by getting into the (gay) parade and all manner of things that I considered quite bold and refreshing."

The final reason for optimism is the recent expansion of the lesbian and gay male subcultures. Groups like the Daughters of Bilitis and the Mattachine Society have been on the scene for decades, providing essential meeting places, legal aid, and encouragement. In the past decade, gay people in the United States have given birth to an expanded movement for self-respect and social change, expressed in more than 2,500 clubs, religious groups, lobbying coalitions, and publications. Older gays have played an important role in these groups, openly and behind the scenes. Since many of them have contributed their money and ideas "from the closet", their contributions have often gone unthanked. Lately, more appreciation is being shown to older gays, and their special needs are being addressed by several researchers and organizers.

While there is a long struggle ahead for securing the rights and happiness of older people, of lesbians and gay men, and of older gays in particular, the current social situation is far better than many older gays dreamed of in their youth. The next generation facing middle and old age is likely to arrive fortified, more confident, with more self-esteem, fully expecting their place in the sun.

For additional information, contact:
> SAGE: Senior Action in a Gay Environment, Inc.
> 487-A Hudson Street
> New York, N. Y. 10014
> Telephone: (212) 741-2247

Created by a coalition of concerned members of the local gay community and professionals in social service and gerontology, SAGE contributes to building a social and cultural community supportive to older gay people.

> NALGG: National Association of Lesbian and Gay Gerontologists
> 3312 Descanso Drive
> Los Angeles, California 90026
> Telephone: (213) 661-3138

> Mariposa Education and Research Foundation
> 186 Spring Street
> New York, N. Y. 10012
> Telephone: (212) 431-3843

This group is preparing a collection of reminiscenses of older lesbians and gay men.

DEALING WITH LOSSES
by Sanford I. Finkel, M. D.

In late life there is more likelihood of physical illness, loss of loved ones, difficulty with movement, and a reduced standard of living due to retirement and inflation. Each person reacts to these losses in his or her own characteristic manner. Those who have responded to earlier life crises by becoming depressed, angry, or irritated are likely to do the same when they are older. Other common emotional and behavioral reactions to stress are confusion, suspiciousness, bitterness, and withdrawal.

Let's take a look at some ways to cope with these problems, starting with a middle-aged man worried that his mother is "growing senile."

Confusion

Mr. Anderson brought his 75-year-old mother, who was agitated and confused, to a hospital emergency room. Mrs. Anderson was able to identify her son and give her name but not her address, phone number, or the date. Mr. Anderson said that his mother had been fine until the previous day, at which time she appeared very tired and complained of diarrhea. Even more disturbing to her son, Mrs. Anderson seemed extremely nervous and absent-minded. Her son feared she was "growing senile."

A medical examination of Mrs. Anderson revealed a fever of 102.0 degrees, a rapid pulse, and a state of mild dehydration. Blood tests showed a low potassium level. During Mrs. Anderson's two hours in the emergency room, she had several loose bowel movements. The doctors diagnosed acute viral gastroenteritis (intestinal flu). Fever, dehydration, and low blood potassium from the flu had brought on Mrs. Anderson's state of agitation and confusion. With proper medical treatment — hospitalization, fluids with potassium replacement, and mild anti-anxiety agents — Mrs. Anderson recovered physically in 48 hours. Within one more day, her mental faculties returned to normal!

Older people are often considered "senile" by those with little understanding of the aging process. Many older people themselves fear growing confused and believe that "senility" is inevitable. It is not! In fact, only 5% of all Americans over the age of 65 have significant confusion. As was the case with Mrs. Anderson, most confusion in late life is caused by treatable medical problems.

Take, for example, reactions to drugs, starting with heart medication. Many older people take medication to improve the rhythm or strength of their heart beat. If not taken in exactly the correct dosage, it can actually impair heart function. Then the brain may not receive the oxygen and nutrients it needs to function properly. For anyone who takes heart medication and later becomes confused, the first order of business is to check with the doctor to see if too much medication has been taken.

Many medications to lower blood pressure can cause a loss of potassium. People with low potassium are more likely to develop confusion. This problem can be avoided by making sure the diet contains potassium-rich foods such as bananas, orange juice and tomato juice.

Sleeping pills and tranquilizers such as Librium and Valium may cause confusion. They are helpful to some people who are anxious or have trouble sleeping, but the dose of sleeping pills or tranquilizers for an elderly person should be less than for a younger person. These drugs should be carefully supervised by a physician and stopped when no longer necessary.

In small amounts alcoholic beverages can be as useful as any tranquilizer for relief of tension. However, the body may not tolerate alcohol to the same degree as it did in earlier years. The older person is much more likely to become confused after a moderate amount of liquor.

Several types of infections are notorious for causing confusion in later life. Pneumonia or any problem with breathing reduces the amount of oxygen that reaches the brain and can cause confusion. Intestinal flu, as in our example with Mrs. Anderson, may cause short-term but serious diarrhea, leading to dehydration or potassium loss. Either of these states may result in confusion; if they occur together, the possibility is much more likely.

As is explained in Chapter 11, maintaining the balance between diet, exercise, and medication is crucial for a person with diabetes mellitus ("high blood sugar"). Confusion may be one result of losing this balance.

The problems mentioned so far can be brought on rather rapidly and treated fairly easily. Confusion and memory loss may also develop and worsen over a long period of time due to serious conditions including vitamin deficiency and malnutrition, depression, pernicious anemia, hypothyroidism, adrenal gland abnormalities, blockage of the spinal fluid at the base of the brain (normal pressure hydrocephalus), benign tumors of the brain, and undiagnosed blood clots in the brain. Several recent studies at major medical centers have indicated that 10 to 20% of people with progressive, chronic memory loss have conditions such as these that can be cured. Another 20 to 25% can be helped by halting the disease process or by preventing certain complications.

Years ago, it was thought that memory loss was caused by hardening of the arteries leading to the brain, but recent evidence reveals that this is so only in 20 to 25% of the cases.

If you notice that you or a friend or relative are becoming confused or developing a memory problem, see a physician for a thorough exam. One clue that a memory problem is beginning is a frequent request for compliments for actions normally taken for granted. For example, a man might expect a great compliment for cleaning out the garage or playing a piano piece he mastered long ago. Another clue may be that the time it takes to get dressed or to do other simple tasks becomes increasingly longer. The individual may show less enthusiasm, creativity, ingenuity, and willingness to try new situations, or there may be an increase in the number of hours of sleep he or she needs each night.

Though people with increasing confusion may act well socially, it is often difficult to understand their train of thought. They may have trouble remembering the comments you have made or the questions you asked. They feel they have to respond, and do so, but often with information which is not directly relevant to the conversation.

When an older person becomes extremely confused and no medical treatment is possible, a crisis in the family begins. For the person to stay at home, there must be a family member or friend willing and able to undertake total responsibility for the person's well-being. A husband or wife often insists on staying with the spouse, even though it means an exhausting day-in, day-out schedule. Sometimes the healthy spouse develops a serious illness and needs to be hospitalized, creating an emergency in terms of the confused loved one. Plans for an alternate living situation then must be made without much preparation or examination of alternatives.

Social service agencies, religious groups, and senior citizen centers have staff who are experienced with such problems and can lend support. An excellent new development is day centers for the elderly.

It is important that the planning for care of the older person allow for the primary care-taker to have a few hours a day to rest or to be with friends.

Depression

Mr. Belom was a 73-year-old successful businessman who continued to work 60 hours a week. He was proud of playing tennis twice a week, and of his mental sharpness. Then he suffered a stroke and developed serious speech and walking problems. He became severely depressed and seriously considered suicide. His wife became frantic. A cardiac patient herself, she developed physical and emotional problems in response to her husband's condition. Mr.

Belom saw a psychiatrist for intensive psychotherapy and anti-depressant medications. He was hospitalized for several days, until he no longer felt suicidal. His wife also saw the psychiatrist once a week. Ultimately, Mr. Belom was able to return to work, though on a more limited basis. Eventually he went on to other recreational activities which met his needs. Physical therapy and speech therapy improved his walking and speaking until they became essentially normal.

Depression such as Mr. Belom faced can be severely disabling. Depression is different from loneliness, which means isolation from the closeness and warmth of human contact. It is also different from grief or mourning, a common response to loss, discussed in the chapter on grieving in this book. Depression includes many of the following: a feeling of hopelessness or apathy, a feeling of pessimism about the future, a sense of worthlessness, inability to stay asleep (early morning awakening), loss of appetite resulting in loss of weight, preoccupation with one's body, feelings of guilt, decreased sexual interest, sluggishness or lack of energy, constipation, loss of customary interests, and feeling very sad during the early morning hours.

Most of the depressions in late life are responses to one or many losses. These losses may be physical, such as a decrease in vision in someone who has been an avid reader, or a loss of close family or friends through death, illness, or moving away. The losses may also be psychological, as in a loss of self esteem brought on by rejection, criticism, or disappointment.

Following a series of losses, the older person may underestimate his or her strengths. One particular strength which may be overlooked is the ability to turn to others who can be helpful during difficult times. Some people feel too proud to ask for help, either of family members or trained mental health professionals. It is especially important to get help when a change in life-style is required, such as after the loss of a spouse or after an illness which limits one's functioning. Anti-depressant medication can also be useful. In recent years, researchers have found evidence that the central nervous systems of most depressed people contains lower than normal levels of certain chemicals called catecholamines. Anti-depressant medications such as Sinequan, Norpramine, Elavil, and Tofranil increase the level of these chemicals.

Some people tend to get very depressed over and over again. Taking a careful history, a physician can often find a family history of such depressions. In recent years, some physicians have effectively used the drug Lithium Carbonate to minimize the impact of these depressions. For people with severe depressions not responsive to the types of treatment already described, electro-convulsive therapy (E. C. T.) may be helpful. This is true only in a small percentage of cases, yet it can be life-saving in people inclined toward suicide and can reduce suffering quickly in others. E. C. T. is stigmatised in our society, probably the result of its overuse in some of the State mental hospitals during the 1930's and 1940's and its misuse by some physicians to this date. However, medications to relax muscles, reduce secretions, and induce sleep make the *appropriate* use of E. C. T. quite safe and effective.

One common form depression may take in later life is hypochondriasis. This is a preoccupation with one's health, including making many physical complaints for which no physical cause can be found. For some people, it is less painful to express unhappiness through bodily complaints than to talk about feelings and disappointments in relation to children, retirement, the loss of loved ones, and other problems.

Untreated depression may cause memory loss and confusion, loss of appetite, poor sleep, and loss of social life. With proper treatment, one's mood, self-image and health improve and intellectual functions return to normal. The vast majority of depressions are treatable.

Paranoid Reactions

Mrs. Carter, a mentally active 88-year-old woman, was always socially isolated. Her great pleasure had been reading, and she always considered herself self-sufficient. As her vision failed, she felt more and more helpless. She had difficulty taking care of the house and shopping for herself. She began to sleep poorly, lose weight, and feel that her end was near. Her state of withdrawal ended suddenly when she began to call the police, accusing her janitor of breaking into her apartment and stealing things. She became very agitated. Brief psychiatric hospitalization was necessary. At the hospital she was diagnosed as having cataracts. Successful surgery on one eye improved her vision. With considerable support from neighbors and a nearby social agency, she was able to return to the community.

Paranoid reactions like Mrs. Carter's are most common in later life. They often develop in response to depression — feeling worthless, helpless, and hopeless. The paranoid person is not aware of these feelings. Instead, the person believes that his or her problems are caused by others. If the people on whom the paranoid person blames his or her problems are far removed — such as the Chinese Communists or business or labor interests — there may be little disruption in functioning. However, if the person under suspicion is a close relative, the situation may quickly reach desperate proportions. Then not only is the paranoid person agitated and fearful, but he or she may also be threatened with the loss of the chief source of human support. One definite advantage of being paranoid, as opposed to being depressed, is that it increases the chances of obtaining professional help. There are many people in the community, for example, who are silently depressed and bother no one. However, when they become paranoid and accuse other prople of creating their problems, they are often referred by neighbors, family, police, or landlords to physicians, mental health professionals, or social agencies.

Paranoid reactions, particularly those that have started recently, are usually treatable. A non-threatening relationship, often with a mental health professional, and small to moderate doses of medication to reduce anxiety usually result in a return to normal functioning. Some people have long histories of severe paranoid reactions as part of serious long-term problems such as schizophrenia. With the right kind of support and medication these people should recover from their acute episodes.

Perceptual Changes

Many older people experience changes in their vision and hearing. In general, a gradual decrease in visual acuity is psychologically managed quite well. Though cataracts and glaucoma gradually impair vision, there is time to compensate and psychologically adjust to this shift. On the other hand, if there is a sudden dramatic loss of vision such as may occur following cataract surgery on one adequate eye, there is a likelihood of a severe psychological reaction. Such a loss is similar to the sensory deprivation which has been reported in prisoner of war camps and outer space travel — it is a sudden absence of normal, everyday perceptual stimulation. Following surgery, this loss is combined with a change in environment and daily schedule. To minimize the likelihood of a severe psychological reaction to such surgery, it would be best to have a familiar person available at the bedside as much as possible. Early discharge from the hospital is also advised.

Other visual changes include the different perception of colors. This is caused by a yellowing of the lens in the eye. For this reason, some older people prefer bright colors. There is also a change in accommodation, which means that it takes longer to adjust to an environment where there is little light, such as a movie theater. Many older people prefer not to dine by candlelight because of this.

Changes in hearing are even more likely than changes in vision to produce psychological stress. If one cannot hear properly, it becomes difficult to understand one's environment. For example, a daughter says to her hard-of-hearing mother, "I'm going to the store now to shop for you. If they will deliver, I'll see you the day after tomorrow. Otherwise, I'll see you tonight with the groceries." If the mother heard the first and third sentences but not the second, she will be expecting her daughter that very night. When the groceries are delivered but the daughter does not come, mother will be angry and disappointed. Repeated misunderstandings with her daughter and others could easily lead this woman into feeling suspicious and misused. In fact, evidence indicates that people with hearing disorders have a higher incidence of paranoia than people with normal hearing.

Hearing loss can also contribute to tension in inter-personal relationships. Because the hard-of-hearing person must talk loudly — sometimes even shout — to hear himself, he may become irritable and socially withdrawn. This, in turn, can lead to suspiciousness or depression. Some hearing disorders can be improved by hearing aids or surgery; others are a result of irreversible nerve death. A thorough diagnostic evaluation is imperative when hearing grows difficult.

Family Problems

Adults and their aging parents want respect, admiration, and affection from each other. This is sometimes quite difficult to work out. The parents have lost people, jobs, and abilities that meant a lot to them. Holding in their negative feelings may lead to depression. But expressing strong emotions to neighbors or friends may frighten them away. It often feels safest to share these pent-up feelings with one's closest relatives.

Adult children usually want to help their parents. Out of love and out of guilt, they listen to their parents and try to be closer and more giving. Although the parents generally appreciate their children's concern and help, they may still feel angry about the many changes in their children. The children may take this frustration personally and become angry. This guilt-help-anger cycle may be repeated for many years. It often helps if parents and children sit down together — perhaps with somebody more objective — and try to listen to each other. Each of us has out own limitations, and life is limited by old age and death; what can we realistically do to appreciate and help ourselves and each other?

Another difficult issue for adult children is what to do when their parents can't take care of themselves. One common notion is that children "dump" their parents into nursing homes. Sometimes the problem is just the opposite — a parent is kept at home beyond an appropriate time. The emotional and physical needs of the family member taking care of an old parent must also be considered. It may be helpful to talk with a skilled social worker or physician about day centers, retirement homes, and nursing homes when close supervision or intensive medical attention is needed.

Retirement

For some, retirement comes as a relief, an end to the obligation to work. It provides an opportunity for reading, hobbies, and more time with family. Twenty percent of retiring men experience an increase in sexual activities, and retirees often improve their health. But retirement may also cause anxiety. It may be associated with a sense of uselessness, loss of identity, and financial hardship. Retirement may also lead to anger at being "dumped" just because one has reached age 62 or 65. Successful retirement depends on one's financial status, health, personality, and opportunities. There is evidence that those people who choose when and how to retire will find more satisfaction and fulfillment than those who have no choice.

"Workaholics" who have cultivated little besides their jobs during their adult lives have the most trouble with retirement. Without working, they feel worthless and may develop depression or more serious emotional problems. Professional assistance may be needed and may be life-saving.

The woman's liberation movement, with its emphasis on changing sex roles, may diminish men's retirement problems. As men participate more actively in household activities, raising the children, and developing leisure activities, it is quite likely that their post-retirement years will be more productive and happy.

Psychological Goals of Later Life

It is very important to look back and find some meaning in the many experiences of one's life. By thinking, talking with friends or family, or writing in a journal it is possible to develop a better understanding of one's self and one's historical development. People loved or hated, jobs, homes, wars, places seen, political events, and personal ups and downs fall into place in each unique life. Problems which may have been disturbing at one phase of the life cycle may now be seen in a different light and be accepted. The successful life-review or reminiscence may lead to a greater sense of wisdom and inner tranquility. It may also bring a frankness and straightforwardness which is less often seen in younger people.

Most people late in life want to feel a sense of continuity with younger people. This may mean telling "one's story" to children or granchildren, sharing the particulars of one life and thoughts on a whole period of history. It may also mean sharing one's knowledge and experience with younger people involved in the same occupation, hobbies, or political concerns. Another way of providing continuity is by making wills, distributing important belongings, and materially assisting younger family members. In all these ways, an older person can have the important feeling of contributing to the younger generations. This is a kind of immortality.

GRIEVING: A NATURAL PART OF LIFE

by Laurieann Chutis

You have just been told that your loved one has died. Your mind screams out, "No, no, this cannot be!"Your body tightens. You find it difficult to breathe. You are stunned by a knowledge that brings no understanding — the person you have lived your life with, your spouse, is no longer alive. Here begins the process called grieving.

Grieving is normal. It is also painful. It affects us both physically and mentally. Grieving takes time, but it follows no schedule. Each person has his or her own timetable for grief and recovery.

Much has been said in the past few years about the emotional and physical stages of dying, but until very recently little has been said about the feelings of the survivors. Now, however, self-help groups for widows and widowers are beginning to spring up across the country. These groups give people a chance to talk openly with others "in the same boat." I have met with more than 150 widows and widowers in Chicago-area groups, and have talked with members of similar groups in other parts of the

country. In this chapter I will share with you what I
have heard, felt, and learned. What I will share is
not a rigid method for grieving, but the range of
experiences people have shared with me. See how
your own experiences are similar or different, and
perhaps you will find in these words the comfort of
knowing you are not alone.

People seem to experience three different stages
or periods of grieving. These are called the shock,
recoil, and recovery stages. Some people move
naturally from one stage to the next. Others stay in
one stage, while still others go from shock to recoil
and back to shock.

Shock. "What? It can't be!" This is the first stage.
Some people express their horror in crying and
screaming, but many others experience a numbness: they cannot believe that the person they love
is dead. They may become unable to speak or think.
"Isn't she holding up well?!" relatives might say at
the funeral. But inside, the survivor is in turmoil.
Some widows and widowers feel guilty at not being
able to cry at the funeral, convinced that not crying
means they did not love their spouse. Nothing could
be further from the truth: numbness and guilt are
simply reactions to the trauma of loss. The survivor
cannot absorb the experience of death, so she pro-
tects herself by becoming numb. A widow may deny
that her husband is dead. In the back of her mind,

she keeps thinking he surely will walk in the door or call to tell her everything is all right.

This shock stage can last from one day to six months, or longer.

Recoil, the second stage, hits with a force that most widows and widowers do not expect. This is the time when the widower begins fully to realize that his wife is dead and will never be back. He feels physical and emotional pain as fresh as if wife had just died. This is the time for crying, for anger at his wife for leaving or at the doctor for letting her die. Now grieving may take its toll physically. Loss of appetite is common, although some people eat non-stop. Many people feel a heaviness in the body and around the heart.

It is natural to relive, retell the events of the death and of the funeral. One's loneliness becomes unbearable. Many people at this point try to finish what is unfinishable — like completing the sweater a woman had started for her husband or painting the room the color he always wanted. Many people blame themselves during this stage for the death of their spouse: "If only I had gotten him/her to the doctor or changed his/her diet, maybe he/she would be alive today." For others, there is a wish to die themselves, to join their spouses. Many people report that they see their spouse sitting in his/her favorite chair, or that they talk to the spouse as if he or she were present in the room.

These feelings are all normal. Recoil is a time of sharp pain and confusion. Many widows and widowers have found it helpful to talk to someone about their feelings and their experiences. Talking doesn't take away the pain, but it does help take the fear and worry out of this very difficult time. Many have found it hard to talk to their relatives and friends about this stage in grieving. Well-meaning people might tell you to "take hold of yourself," to "get involved in new activities," that "the time for grieving is over." Only you can decide that for yourself. If you need to cry, if you need to talk, if you need to remember, do it! Find someone who understands. Find a group or a person, another widow or widower who can hear your pain, who can sit there with you and listen. Some people need to do their crying alone. Yet most widows and widowers feel better when they discuss their experiences with people who understand. They get satisfaction from knowing that they are not crazy, that they are not alone.

Recovery, the third stage, begins in many different ways. It may be the first time you wake up and the first thought in your head is *not* that your husband or wife is dead. It may be the first time you laugh and then feel guilty that you laughed. It may be the first time you begin thinking about living, living now as a widow or widower, not as a wife or husband. Recovery does not mean forgetting. One always remembers, sometimes with pain, sometimes with joy.

This is the time when you begin making decisions about how you will live out your life, and these decisions must be made without your spouse being there to help. How will you live with loneliness? Should you look for new activities and new friends, or go back to old friends and old activities? Most people do experiment during this time. They will try a new activity and maybe decide that it is not for them and try out something else. For most people it takes time, time to decide what feels right.

Friends and relatives all give advice on how they want you to be. Only you will know what's right for you. You are a person. You are a person who has lost your spouse. But above all, you are a person and have a right to live your life as you see fit.

Part of recovery is making financial and legal decisions. Get information on your spouse's pension and the Will. See what help you can get from Social Security, Public Aid, the Veterans Administration, or senior citizens' groups. Talk to the family lawyer or see someone at a local legal aid clinic. Talk to a widow/widower organization in your community.You'll meet people who have had to make decisions very similar to the ones you are making right now.

One of the most important decisions that widows/widowers make is the question of living alone or living with their adult children. There are advantages and disadvantages to both. Remaining in the same house or apartment, you are constantly reminded of the time when your spouse was there. If you are now living alone, there are problems of dealing with aloneness and loneliness. Yet this place is familiar to you. You know your neighbors, the grocery store, the bus, street, your church.

Many widows and widowers wish to leave their home and neighborhood and move in with their children. They want their children to help them financially and emotionally. They don't want to be alone. They find value in being involved in the lives of their children. But others do not like "being a burden" to their children, having to adjust to their children's lifestyle, losing their old friends and neighbors. They find it difficult to make new friends. Many say they find that they are just as lonely with a roomful of grandchildren as they were in their own home alone.

Some people who decided quickly to sell their homes and move in with their children have regretted that they did not give themselves more time to think it over. They suggest that it is better, if you can afford it, to maintain your own living quarters and to experiment with other lifestyles. For instance, you might have a friend come stay with you for a couple of months. If you enjoy that arrangement, you may decide to have a roomer or a companion move in with you. You might want to visit your adult children and see how living with them feels for you. Just as the grieving process takes time, major decisions take time. Today it might be unbearable to live in an empty house or apartment. Tomorrow you may appreciate the independence and freedom you have in being alone.

One of the most important things widows and widowers say they can do for themselves during this time of grief is to reach out for support when they need it. Support can come in terms of information regarding the will, pensions, and financial survival. It can come from joining a senior citizen meal program for hot food and friends. Support can be someone willing to listen to your tears, confusion, and pain. For many widows and widowers their children, church, old friends, and neighbors provide a great deal of this emotional support, but others have found that their children cannot provide what they need. The children are experiencing their own grief over the loss of a parent. Sometimes old friends and neighbors have their own opinions on how you should be or act as a widow or widower. They may become uncomfortable with your strong emotions and urge you to "shape up."

Finally, support can come from organizations made up of surviving spouses. For many it is very helpful to talk to another widow or widower who has "been there."

You can talk to a widow to get her advice, to understand how she's made it through the grieving process, how she's survived and what meaning life has for her now. There is a phone service where you can be called on an ongoing basis to talk over how you are doing. There are rap groups, discussion groups, lectures that you can attend to hear how others have worked through their grief. There are groups that are formed for social activities, for widows/widowers to go out together to plays and dinners with new friends who can accept you whether you're feeling happy or needing to cry.

If you are interested, take a risk and call a widow/widower group.Get information about the meetings. If the group interests you, try it out. If you don't like it, you don't have to go.

Remember, you are not alone. There are 250,000 widowers and ten million widows in the United States, and 75% of them are over 65 years of age. It is normal to experience confusion, pain, and loneliness. You are doing the important work of grieving. For many people the stages of shock, recoil, and recovery take at least two years. Give yourself time to grieve. Give yourself time to learn what you enjoy, and time to make decisions.

As the weeks and months go by, you make the choices that seem right for you. You make decisions, one by one. You define what it means to be you. By yourself, and with others, you rediscover life.

For further information:

Job Finding Techniques for Mature Women
Superintendent of Documents
U. S. Government Printing Office
Washington, D. C. 20402
(enclose 30¢)

Widow to Widow Program Kit
Harvard Medical School
Laboratory of Community Psychiatry
Boston, Massachusetts 01115
(enclose $2.50)

MASSAGE — IT'S NICE TO BE KNEADED

by Robert K. King

A few years ago I was visiting my grandmother in an old-age home just outside of Chicago. As we sat and talked in the hospitality room, I was struck by the conversation of several of her friends who were complaining of irregularity, headaches, recent surgery, swelling in the feet, migraine headaches, shortness of breath, and aching joints. I asked four people in the room to stop talking about their ailments for a few minutes and simply to close their eyes, sit comfortably, and relax. Then I gave each of them what I call a "tune-up treatment" — a good massage of the shoulder, head, and neck.

In less than 20 minutes, the change was unbelievable! The four people appeared calm. The pinched looks on their faces had vanished. Their skin appeared softer. Their breathing was deeper. They all commented on how good they felt. A sense of relaxation and well-being was in the air. My grandmother later told me that for the rest of the day she and her friends were happier than usual.

This didn't surprise me. All people have a profound need to be touched in a nurturing fashion. Frequent complaining comes partly from not being touched enough. Massage can contribute to calmness and self-esteem.

For some time, massage had a bad reputation. It was considered a luxury of the rich at expensive beauty spas. Or people thought of it as a sexual treatment provided at "massage parlors." Some thought massage was only for individuals with chronic health problems such as bad backs, arthritis or muscle spasms. Fortunately, people are now broadening their thinking on the nature and possible benefits of massage.

For good reason! You can expect several pleasurable benefits from regular massage treatments. The main result is a lessening of tension throughout the body. Such tension interferes with blood circulation, reduces energy, makes deep breathing difficult, and drastically reduces enthusiasm for life. With massage, our bodies become more relaxed and our minds more positive.

Medical doctors frequently prescribe massage for a wide variety of ailments among older people, such as arthritis, insomnia, constipation, edema, nervous tics, and paralysis. Naturally, you should check with your physician if you have any serious problems before starting either professional or do-it-yourself massage treatments. It could be dangerous, for example, to receive a massage if you have an unstable heart condition, a history of blood clots in your veins (thrombophlebitis), an unexplained pain in your calf, severe varicose veins, tuberculosis, a tendency to bleed easily (hemorrhage), open sores, a rash, or a contagious fever.

As a matter of professional ethics, the competent massage practitioner will never try to diagnose disease. If you are in good health but suffering from minor aches and pains, then a prescription for massage is not necessary.

Some professional masseurs overstate the benefits of massage in order to drum up more business. They often direct their pitches at older people using three popular myths, each of which has a kernel of truth to it. Here is the real story:

First, massage does not reduce weight. It does not "break up" accumulations of fatty tissue. Diet and exercise are the ways to lose weight. By relaxing the muscles and improving circulation, however, massage can improve your appearance.

Second, massage will not eliminate wrinkles. As a person grows older, up to 50% of his or her muscular tissue is lost. The muscle is replaced by fat which does not take up as much room or have the same firmness. It just sits there, covered by wrinkled and loose skin. If you want to keep more muscle, then exercise more. What massage can do is help keep your skin soft and healthy and help give your face a more relaxed and pleasant look.

Third, massage does not take the place of regular exercise. It does not replace walking, swimming, or dancing. It is, however, often prescribed as a form of "passive exercise" for individuals who cannot actively engage in various physical exercises and activities. For example, an arm may be massaged and moved through its entire range of motion by a friend of someone who has a weak arm due to a stroke. Massage can loosen and relax your muscles and joints and relieve some of the stiffness of arthritis.

Let's say you would like to get a good professional massage treatment. What are some guidelines to follow?

1. Get a word-of-mouth referral from a friend who is already enjoying the benefits of massage, or check the credentials of the practitioner.

2. Check the surroundings to be sure they are clean and sanitary.

3. Discuss any medical problems and pains with the massage practitioner before you receive a treatment. In this way, the practitioner will know whether to give you a massage, what areas of your body to focus on, and what approach to take.

4. Be your own judge regarding the length of the treatment. Many people limit themselves to 20 or 30 minutes to avoid feeling tired.

5. Never endure a treatment which leaves you with bruises or a sense of exhaustion. Tell the person working on you if too much pressure is being used at any time during the treatment.

6. Remember, you don't have to wait to be stiff or sore to get a good massage. Regular treatments can help you preserve a sense of feeling healthy.

Would you like to learn the "tune-up treatment" I mentioned in telling the story about my grandmother? You can practice this technique with your friends even if you have no experience in massage. It is easy to perform and soothing to receive. If you have two interested friends, all the better. One can read the instructions, another give the "tune-up," and the third lucky one get "worked on." Then you can trade roles.

While you are giving your friend the treatment, occasionally close your eyes and "let your hands do the thinking." Experiment with the amount of pressure you use. Listen to any feedback from your partner regarding which strokes feel especially good or bad. You don't need cream, oil or a specially designed treatment table. Any low-backed comfortable chair will do.

Start by having your partner sit straight but comfortably in a chair, closing his or her eyes and relaxing. Have your friend take three nice sighs, shrug the shoulders, and wiggle into a comfortable position.

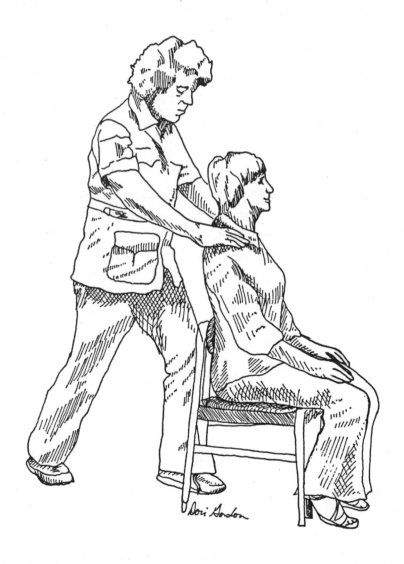

Stand behind your partner and knead the two muscles on either side of the neck next to the shoulders. These trapezius muscles are frequently tense like ropes. Start with very little pressure, then squeeze harder.

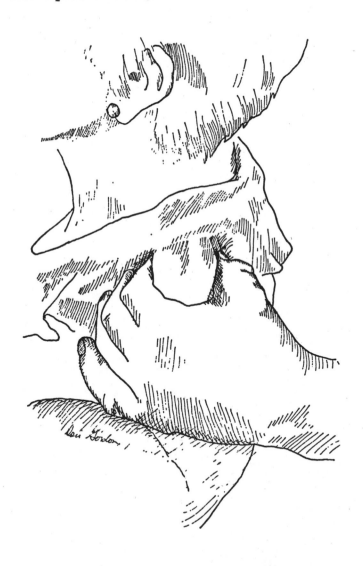

Next go to the back of the neck. Support your friend's forehead with one of your hands. With the thumb and first two fingers of your other hand, make tiny circles at the base of the skull. Be sure to support the forehead firmly. This lets your partner's neck muscles relax from their work of supporting the head, weighing between 10 and 12 pounds! Gently squeeze the entire back of the neck.

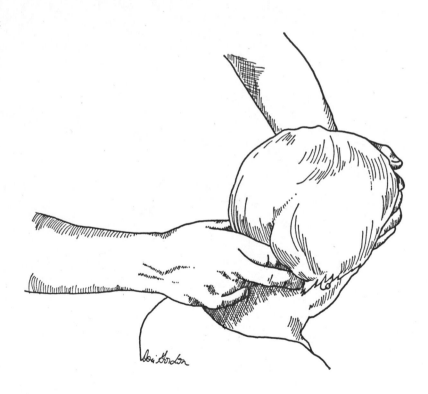

Lift the head up again. Spread the fingers of both of your hands and make a light "scissors motion" over the entire scalp, as though you are working up a shampoo lather. This technique is especially good for relieving tension headaches. If you do it for three or four minutes in a nurturing way, your partner will probably become very relaxed and pleasantly drowsy.

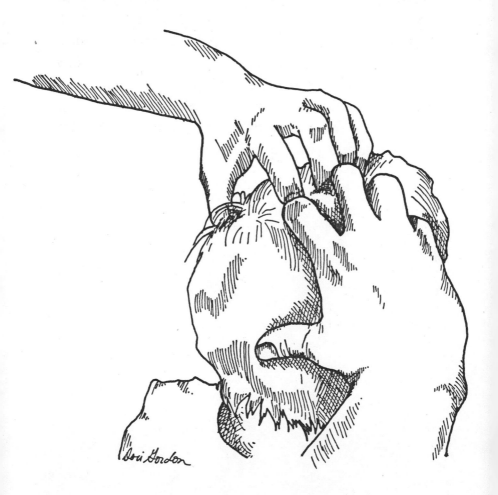

Now use a very light scratching motion all over the scalp and around the temples. Close your eyes as you are stroking your partner's entire scalp, and go slowly. From time to time, take a nice deep breath yourself. The more you relax, the more your friend relaxes.

Move to the upper back and shoulders again, kneading lightly. Take a step to the right and massage the right shoulder and upper arm, moving back to the neck. Imagine you are kneading dough for bread, using both hands and squeezing. Now step to the left and proceed with the same technique on your friend's left shoulder and upper arm. Try leaning into the movements, so that your body does more work and your hands do less.

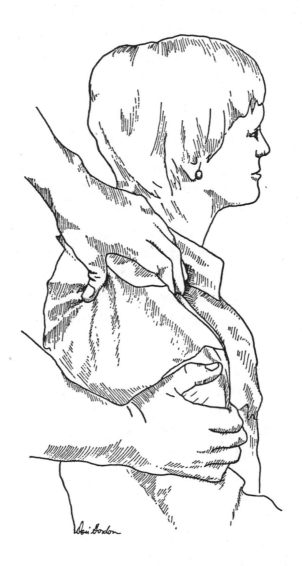

Next, use a "thumb crawling" technique. Press both thumbs down, one on each shoulder. The move them up pressing firmly at half-inch intervals until both thumbs reach the neck at the same time. Can you feel that muscle like a rope or rubber tube under the skin? Repeat this movement four or five times. By not spending too much time on one particular technique, your hands will not get tired.

Pick up your tempo slightly and knead alongside the upper back, shoulders and upper arms, starting with one hand at either side of the neck. As you knead, you are actually grasping, squeezing and releasing in a rapid fashion, being careful not to pinch or gouge. You work your hands away from one another, ending at the upper arms. Then reverse the process by massaging back to either side of the neck.

Now let your hands rest on your partner's shoulders. Breathe. End the massage by sending a feeling of friendship through your hands, letting them rest on your friend's shoulders for a moment, and slowly letting your hands drop to your side. The entire "tune-up treatment" will last about 10 minutes. If you like to do it longer, fine! As you give and receive massages more frequently, you will notice yourself developing a better sense of touch. You will be able to feel the difference between tense areas and relaxed areas and develop a good notion of

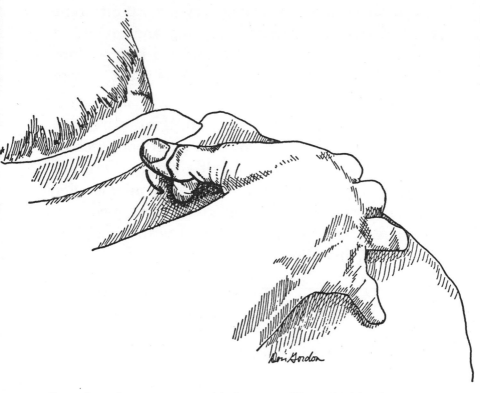

how hard to squeeze. And you will probably discover a favorite way you like to be massaged.

When you are receiving a massage, sit as comfortably as possible. Breathe easily and imagine that your muscles are becoming soft in your friend's hands. Enjoy the attention, the touching, the nurturing. Feel free to say "too hard", "too soft", or "more of that."

Listening to this kind of feedback is an excellent way to improve your massage skills. You could, for example, have a friend remove his/her shirt and lie face down on a bed or couch. Try several different ways of gently and firmly stroking and squeezing your friend's back. The comments you hear — "not so hard," "slower, please," "that feels great" — are your guidelines.

For some, massage can be an excellent retirement skill. If you want to learn some additional techniques and develop your touching skills, there are amateur and professional courses available. For almost anyone at any age, giving and receiving massages can enrich day-to-day life with friendship, relaxation, and pleasure.

For more information, see *The Massage Book*, by George Downing. New York: Random House — Bookworks, 1972. This is one of the finest books available for clear, illustrated massage guidelines.

SMOOTH TO THE TOUCH ON TOP
by Robert J. Skeist, R. N.

On his Baldness

At dawn I sighed to see my hairs fall;
  At dusk I sighed to see my hairs fall.
For I dreaded the time when the last lock should
  go...
  They are all gone and I do not mind at all!
I have done with that cumbrous washing and
  getting dry;
  My tiresome comb for ever is laid aside.
Best of all, when the weather is hot and wet,
  To have no top-knot weighing down on one's head!
I put aside my dusty conical cap;
  And loose my collar-fringe.
In a silver jar I have stored a cold stream;
  On my bald pate I trickle a ladle-full.
Like one baptizer with the Water of Buddha's Law,
  I sit and receive this cool, cleansing joy.
Now I know why the priest who seeks Repose
  Frees his heart by first shaving his head.

On the phone with John Callahan of the *Weekly Review,* Chicago's senior citizen newspaper, I mentioned my plans for writing about the positive side of balding. John at 52 and I at 31 are both quite smooth to the touch on top. He was thrilled with my idea. John pulled from his bookshelf Arthur Waley's *Translations From the Ancient Chinese* and read to me the above delightful poem, written by our brother Po Chu-i in the year 832 C. E.

The negative side of balding is well-known: embarrassment, anxiety about looking old, fear of losing sex-appeal, countless crude jokes. The worst time comes when much of the top hair has departed and one combs a few lonely strands up and over. What if the wind blows the wrong way?

Now I would not consider trying to hide my baldness. Quite the opposite. I lather up and shave on top, removing a few frizzy patches, and keep the remaining horseshoe of hair trimmed and healthy. As our Chinese friend indicated over a thousand years ago, a bald man spends less time shampooing, drying and combing than does his hairy counterpart. May I share with you, especially my bald comrades of all ages, a few more benefits?

Lightly stroking the top of my head helps me think. It has led to at least as many writing ideas as has stroking my beard.

Also, a nice tan. Better than any other part of my body, my bald head soaks up the sun rays.

Finally, we bald men are the connoisseurs of head massage. A back rub is nice, yes. And shoulders enjoy a good kneading. But there's something quite special about having a friend place a drop or two of moisturizer on my smooth pate and rub it in with firm circular movements of the fingertips — a sensual delight for both of us, a great expression of love.

SURVIVING THE MEDICAL SYSTEM

PATIENTS HAVE RIGHTS!
by Robert Skeist, R. N.

It is not written on parchment, but printed on paper. It is not signed by the Founding Fathers, but by hospital administrators. Most people never heard of it, although the Gray Panthers visited every hospital in Cincinnati to see that it was prominently displayed. It is one of the best-kept secrets of modern medicine — *The Patients' Bill of Rights*.

Approved by the American Hospital Association in 1973, this document affirms your right to informed consent, privacy, information about alternative treatments, and "above all, the recognition of (your) dignity as a human being." Here is the full text (emphasis added):

The American Hospital Association presents a Patient's Bill of Rights with the expectation that observance of these rights will contribute to more effective patient care and greater satisfaction for the patient, his physician, and the hospital organization.

1. The patient has the right to considerate and respectful care.

2. The patient has the right to complete current *information concerning his diagnosis, treatment,*

and prognosis in terms the patient can be reasonably expected to *understand*. When it is not medically advisable to give such information to the patient, the information should be made available to an appropriate person in his behalf. He has the right to know by name the physician responsible for coordinating his care.

3. The patient has the right to receive from his physician information necessary to give *informed consent* prior to the start of any procedure and/or treatment. Except in emergencies, such information for informed consent should include but not necessarily be limited to the *specific procedure* and/or treatment, the medically significant *risks* involved, and the probable duration of incapacitation. Where medically significant *alternatives for care* or treatment exist, or when the patient requests information concerning medical alternatives, the patient has the right to such information. The patient also has the right to know the name of the person responsible for the procedures and/or treatment.

4. The patient has the right to *refuse treatment* to the extent permitted by law, and to be informed of the medical consequences of his action.

5. The patient has the right to every consideration of his *privacy* concerning his own medical care program. Case discussion, consultation,

examination, and treatment are confidential and should be conducted discreetly. Those not directly involved in his care must have the permission of the patient to be present.

6. The patient has the right to expect that all communications and *records* pertaining to his care should be treated as *confidential.*

7. The patient has the right to expect that within its capacity a hospital must make *reasonable response to the request of a patient for services.* The hospital must provide evaluation service, and/or referral as indicated by the urgency of the case. When medically permissible a patient may be transferred to another facility only after he has received complete information and explanation concerning the needs for an alternatives to such a transfer. The institution to which the patient is to be transferred must first have accepted the patient for transfer.

8. The patient has the right to obtain information as to any relationship of his hospital to other health care and educational institutions insofar as his care is concerned. The patient has the right to obtain information as to the existence of any professional relationships among individuals, by name, who are treating him.

9. The patient has the right to be advised if the hospital proposes to engage in or perform *human experimentation* affecting his care or

treatment. The patient has the *right to refuse* to participate in such research projects.

10. The patient has the right to expect reasonable *continuity of care.* He has the right to know in advance what appointment times and physicians are available and where. The patient has the right to expect that the hospital will provide a mechanism whereby he is informed by his physician or a delegate of the physician of the patient's *continuing health care requirements following discharge.*

11. The patient has the right to examine and receive an *explanation of his bill* regardless of source of payment.

12. The patient has the right to know what *hospital rules and regulations* apply to his conduct as a patient.

No catalogue of rights can guarantee for the patient the kind of treatment he has a right to expect. A hospital has many functions to perform, including the prevention and treatment of disease, the education of both health professionals and patients, and the conduct of clinical research. All these activities must be conducted with an overriding concern for the patient, and *above all, the recognition of his dignity as a human being.* Success in achieving this recognition assures success in the defense of the rights of the patient.

The National League for Nursing has published a similar list of rights, as have other professional and consumer organizations. Important court rulings have thrown the weight of law behind several specific rights, including the responsibility of hospitals to provide you with good physical and mental care, your right to access to your own medical records, and your physician's responsibility to obtain your informed consent before performing any surgery.

Imagine Estelle Johnson, a 58-year-old woman who has just come out of the shower and is doing her monthly breast examination. She finds a lump the size of a lima bean. She goes to her doctor, who asks her to come into the hospital "so we can take a look at the lump and see if it is malignant." She signs in. Soon a nurse brings her a form to sign, granting permission to the surgeon to perform a "left breast biopsy with possible radical mastectomy."

Mrs. Johnson does not yet sign the form. She politely but firmly asks to see the surgeon. When he arrives, she asks him the meaning of "with possible radical mastectomy." The surgeon explains that he is seeking her permission to examine a piece of the breast lump and then do as much surgery as he thinks is necessary, which could include removal of a breast. "Is there another way to go about this?" Mrs. Johnson asks. There is. She can grant permission now only for the biopsy. If the tests then show that the lump is malignant, she can then discuss with her doctor the full range of alternatives, including removal of part of the breast, radiation therapy, and removal of the entire breast. Mrs. Johnson decides to agree now only to the biopsy. The phrase "with possible radical mastectomy" is struck from the consent form. She signs the form. She prepares herself mentally for the surgery, knowing that she will emerge from the operating room with her breast still there. Estelle Johnson is exercising her right as a patient to receive relevant information and then give her informed consent.

Or picture David Silverstein, age 67, who is annoyed day and night by low back pain. His doctor recommends bed rest and aspirin. Still the back aches. Mr. Silverstein visits another doctor, an orthopedic surgeon, who recommends surgery. This sounds rather drastic. So our friend, on a long shot, goes to one more doctor, a woman who had addressed his senior citizens' group on holistic health. She examines Mr. Silverstein, asks him dozens of questions, and finds that he is willing to take an active role in his own recovery. She suggests he sleep on a firm mattress, do twenty minutes of stretching and strengthening exercises each morning and evening, and take a warm shower daily. Slowly but steadily, over the next six months, his back improves. David Silverstein is exercising his right as a patient to learn of "medically significant alternatives of care."

The medical system often seems mysterious, rushed, and uncaring to the average person seeking help. A doctor may seem too busy for you to "bother" with questions about your condition. A nurse may appear annoyed if you insist on a description of the medicine in the syringe as she aims a needle at your backside. But speak up, as Mrs. Johnson and Mr. Silverstein do. We are talking about *your* body, *your* health, *your* rights.

You Are Not Alone

It is easier to speak up for your rights as a patient when you realize you have support.

1. *Read the "Patients' Bill of Rights" before your next visit to a doctor or hospital.* Remember, these are rights acknowledged by hospital administrators.

2. *Use your doctor and your assigned nurse as resources.* If you have a complaint about the care you are getting, a desire for a different type of food, a question about anything special you should do after you are discharged, or a need for something to be explained in a language other than English, they should be able to answer your question or see that you talk with other relevant staff.

It is important, while you assert your rights, to show respect for hospital workers who serve you. Nurses' aides, physical therapists, transport staff, nurses, and other staff work hard. Like other working people, they often feel powerless, pushed around, unappreciated. Your consideration for them encourages theirs for you. You may find that your nurse or another staff member is delighted to act as your advocate.

3. *If you have problems understanding or asserting your rights, ask if the institution employs an ombudsman to respond to patient complaints.* If not, then ask to see a social worker or a representative of the administration.

4. *Ask a trusted friend or relative to keep in touch with you.* You will probably feel more at ease, and you might get better care, if your support person is with you as you sign in; meets your doctor, your nurse, and the head nurse; gets the phone number of the nurses' station; and visits you regularly. If you have trouble getting important questions answered, a phone call from your support person to your doctor or nurse may help.

5. *In an extreme case, consult a lawyer.* It is clearly preferable to resolve a conflict involving patients' rights by the four alternatives listed

above. Yet occasionally there is an incident of such obvious neglect or malpractice — such as giving an incorrect medication to a basically healthy 60-year-old man that results in his death, or performing medical experiments upon an older welfare recipient without her knowledge — that a lawsuit is justified. Some lawsuits are also valuable in forcing the courts to clarify issues of patients' rights relevant to all of us.

A medical malpractice case is difficult to win and generally requires the talents of a specialist. An effective lawsuit can cost a doctor, a nurse, or a hospital a lot of time and money and could greatly damage a reputation. Be sure that such an extreme action is justified before starting a suit.

Help Them Help You

No doctor, nurse, clinic, or hospital can "make you well" as you just sit back passively. Healing requires your active participation. Here are four ways for you to get the most out of each encounter with the medical system:

1. *Describe how you feel and what you notice about yourself.* Mention pain, fever, constipation, dizziness, depression, and any other problems. This is not being self-indulgent or whiney. Rather, it is giving the medical staff "clues"

for the "detective work" of understanding your condition.

2. *Ask questions.* If you do not understand your illness or treatment, ask your doctor, nurse, pharmacist, and other staff to explain. If the explanation is too complicated, or in technical language you do not understand, ask for a restatement in "plain English."

3. *Take an initiative.* If you are in a hospital and want a specific kind of food (Kosher, vegetarian, etc.), ask to speak with a dietician. If you are recovering from a broken leg or from a stroke and feel ready for exercises, ask your doctor and nurse about starting physical therapy. Before you are discharged from a hospital or end a visit to a clinic or doctor's office, talk with the staff to work out your home plan of diet, exercises, medications, and use of medical equipment.

4. *Follow the treatment plan, or openly contest it.* This means taking medications exactly as directed, sticking to a diet for diabetics, avoiding salt if you have high blood pressure, or following whatever instructions you are given. If you disagree with the advice you are getting or you think that you cannot follow it, it is very important to let your doctor know. The next step will be working out a treatment plan that

both you and your doctor can live with. It is also important that you report any unexpected changes in your condition.

What about Rights in Nursing Homes?

Contrary to the popular notion that at age 65 you get your Medicare card, public transportation discount, and admission ticket to a nursing home, 95% of people 65 and over in the United States live independently in the community. But what of the rights of those in nursing homes? Across the country, people are waking up to the importance of this issue.

The Illinois Nursing Home Care Reform Act of 1979 established a Bill of Rights for nursing home residents. It mandated visiting hours from 10:00 A. M. to 8:00 P. M., secure storage of personal belongings, bank accounts to be provided for residents in possession of $100.00 or more, and the establishing of residents' advisory councils in each home. In other states, similar laws have been passed or are now being considered.

Dr. Robert N. Butler, director of the Naitonal Institute on Aging in Washington, D. C. and a leading advocate for the respectful treatment of our society's elders, urges the creation of watchdog committees composed of nursing home residents, members of their families, and concerned community representatives. In some cities, representatives of senior citizens' groups invite people to let them know of incidents of mistreatment of nursing home residents. A visit to the administrator from members of the seniors' group may then lead to positive results. Nurses connected with the Gray Panthers have prepared a guide for making nursing home reforms.

Last Rights

I took a walk with Anna, a woman in her eighties. Her pace was slow but steady. She told me proudly that her blood pressure was normal, that she had no diabetes and "just a touch of arthritis," that she had never been hospitalized. "True," she said, "my eyes are going, I keep my teeth in a jar at night, I can't keep up the house like I used to, but I'm not doing bad for such a young girl."

Her clubs, her family ties, and reasonable diet and exercise habits helped keep her going, and she seemed as satisfied with life as do most of my friends fifty or sixty years her junior. Yet she spoke as though serious disease might befall her just around the corner.

"You know what really scares me, Robbie?" Anna said, ending a ten-minute silence. "Not dying. Eventually, even if I live to be a hundred, I'll die. I know that, and what can I do? Nothing. I'm old, I'm getting tired, maybe I'm even ready. What scares me is being sick for a long time, in a hospital with tubes stuck in all parts of my body, in pain and helplessness. I want to live at home as long as possible. My daughter said she would stay with me if I needed her. After that, I hope they'll all let me die."

My friend is not alone in her strong feelings. Last summer I sat on the New Jersey beach and spoke with my parents' friend Isidore. He did most of the talking. Generally "strong and silent," his face reddened with anger and tears flowed behind his sunglasses as he described his wife Eunice's last weeks.

Eunice and Isadore were enjoying life together after his retirement. She had her books, he his fishing, they their summer house. I would have guessed they had 15 to 25 years left together. Then came the doctor's report that Eunice had cancer of the pancreas, spreading wildly throughout her abdomen. Fear, pain, hospitals and death followed.

His wife's death infuriated Isadore. There was no "sense" to it. But the behavior of her doctors and hospitals made it all worse. When doctors learned that Eunice had only weeks to live, they broke the news to Isidore in the unprotective setting of a bustling hospital lobby. When Isidore and his psychologist daughter sought information on the latest treatment plans for Eunice, they had to rely on a few concerned nurses and one young intern passing information to them without the doctor's knowledge. When Isidore could tell from the look in

Eunice's eyes that she needed more pain medication, the doctors said no, they did not want her to
become addicted, she would have to wait. "She was
dying, for God's sake!" Isidore shouted at me. "Why
not let her be as comfortable as possible?"

Isidore had asked his doctors about finding a
hospice for his wife. The word "hospice" comes from
the place in medieval times that provided a shelter
for travellers on difficult journeys. More recently,
in England, hospices have been established to allow
dying people to live out their days in as little pain
and with as much respect and love as possible.
Isidore's doctor was annoyed even to be asked about
this kind of care. So this determined man sought the
help of sympathetic nurses, made calls, did
research, and eventually took his wife home. He
bathed her, medicated her, loved her. During her
last few days, when Eunice's pain was so great that
she required a constant flow of medications into her
veins, her husband took her back into the hospital.
Finally the doctors gave her enough medication.
With her family there, she died.

It need not have been so difficult, for Eunice or
for Isidore.

In recent years, experiences such as theirs have
moved seniors' groups, healers, clergy, psychologists, government officials, lawyers and others
to work on the sister issues of hospice and death
with dignity. A network of hospices now exists,

where people who are terminally ill live in home-like centers with natural bedrooms, pets, and family visitors. In many hospices, there is a policy of giving enough medication to really relieve pain and free the residents' attention for other matters. Emotional and spiritual support are emphasized. "Hospice" may also refer to a network of people and services that can help seriously ill people remain in their own homes more comfortably.

"Death with dignity" should be available to everyone, as an alternative to being hospitalized, "stuck with all those tubes," and faced with a prolonged, uncomfortable wait for death. Several states (California, Arkansas, Idaho, Nevada, New Mexico, North Carolina, Oregon, and Texas) have passed "Natural Death" legislation, giving legal recognition to "The Living Will" and similar documents. One version of this will, to be signed by a person in sound mind, is a formal request to physicians, clergy, and family members that *I be allowed to die and not be kept alive by artificial means or heroic measures.*"

"Death is as much a reality as birth, growth, maturity, and old age," the Living Will continues. "It is the one certainty. I do not fear death as much as I fear the indignity of deterioration, dependence, hopeless pain. I ask that drugs be mercifully administered to me for relief of terminal suffering even if they hasten the moment of death."

As affirmed in the Patients' Bill of Rights, the basis of our relationship to the health care system from birth to death must be, above all, the recognition of our dignity as human beings.

For information concerning hospices, contact the National Hospice Organization, 3520 Prospect St., N. W. , No. 336, Washington, D. C. 20007. (203) 338-4733.

For a copy of "Questions and Answers about the Living Will," contact Concern for Dying, 250 W. 57th St., New York, N. Y. 10019

For more general information, see "The Rights of Older Persons," an American Civil Liberties Handbook by Robert N. Brown. New York: Avon Books, 1979.

For additional readings related to patients' rights see interviews in this book with Robert N. Butler, M. D. and Maggie Kuhn, and references following those interviews.

UNDERSTANDING MEDICAL LANGUAGE

by Leo Schlosberg

If your doctor examines you and says you have a case of idiopathic axillary pruritus, don't be alarmed. It means only that your doctor cannot figure out why you have an itchy armpit!

Medical people often use words we do not understand. They learn these words during their training, and later use them in communicating both with other health workers and with us. While it's not a distinctly different language in the way that Italian is, medical terminology is largely foreign to non-medical people. Some of the words have concise equivalents in plain English (axilla = armpit), while others do not (fabella = bones or certain cartilages which may develop in the large leg muscle). Some words, like "appendix," are now part of common, non-technical, English; others, like "fibroblast," are not.

There are a number of ways to get around the language barrier. Medical people can choose to speak to us clearly and give us simple explanations of what they think and what they are doing. It is a pleasure to deal with a doctor or nurse who talks to us about our health and our illness in an understandable manner. But what can we do when medical personnel use technical words that we do not understand?

We can ask for an explanation in plain English. Most of the time the ideas behind the fancy words are not so complicated. It's true that we often feel that medical people are very busy and do not have the time to go explaining everything to us. But the task of medicine is not simply technical — diagnosing and curing us as if we were pieces of machinery — and our needs to know and understand what is going on within us are important. The medical professions exist and are paid to help and to serve *us*. All of us are valuable and important, and matters involving our health should be explained to us by the professionals, no matter how busy they seem to be.

It may sometimes be necessary to point out that medical staff are being paid to do a job which includes giving us clear explanations. Whether we pay them directly or indirectly through insurance or Medicare does not matter. Another approach, if the situation allows it, is to simply change doctors. As more and more of us demand clear information about our health, the medical system will change.

There may be situations in which you will want to find out for yourself the meaning of medical words. Your doctor may not be fluent enough in English to explain your condition to you clearly, or you may be under so much physical and emotional stress that you do not remember the explanation given to you. I recommend purchase of an inexpensive pocket dictionary written especially for non-medical people, such as *The New American Medical Dictionary and Health Manual,* by Robert E. Rothenberg, published by Signet. In 1979, its cost was only $2.50. A more thorough dictionary, commonly used by nurses, is *Taber's Cyclopedic Medical Dictionary,* by Clarence W. Taber, published by F. A. Davis Co. Its price in 1979 was $12.95. *Taber's* does more than define words. It includes information on the causes and symptoms and treatments of diseases. Medical dictionaries are available for public use in public libraries and in most hospital libraries.

Building Medical Words

Many medical words are formed by putting together prefixes (word beginnings), roots (main words), and suffixes (word endings). Knowing a small number of these word parts helps you understand a much larger number of combined words. For example, a common suffix related to surgery is "ectomy" (cut out or remove). A root meaning womb or uterus is "hyster", so "hysterectomy" means removal of the uterus. Similarly, "appendectomy" means removal of the appendix. A good way to learn new medical terms is to guess their meaning from their word parts, then check a medical dictionary. Below is a selected list of prefixes, roots, and suffixes with their definitions and examples of how they combine to form medical words.

Prefix	Meaning	Example
a, an	not, away, without	+esthesis (feeling) = anesthetic (substance that causes one to be without sensation or feeling)
ante	before	+brachium (arm) = antebrachium (forearm)
anti	against	+ coagulant (blood clotting) = anticoagulant (prevents blood clotting)
ecto	external, out, away	+cornea (surface of the eyeball) = ectocornea (outerlayer of the cornea)
endo	into, within	+cardia (heart) = endocardial (within the heart)
exo	outer, away, outside	+ophthal (of the eye) = exophthalmia (bulging out of the eye)
hyper	over, above, more, excessive	+tension (pressure) = hypertension (high blood pressure)

hypo	under, below, less	+derm (skin) = hypodermic needle (needle that goes under the skin)
intra	within	+ocular (eyes) = intraocular pressure (fluid pressure within eyeball)
para	near, beside, around, abnormal	+thyroid = parathyroid (gland located near the thyroid gland)
peri	around	+cardia (heart = pericardium (near the heart; membrane around the heart)
poly	many	+neur (nerve) + algia (pain) = polyneuralgia (pain along many nerves)
pre	before	+operation = pre-operative (before an operation)
pro	before, in front, forward	+thrombin (clotting agent) = prothrombin (chemical in blood from which thrombin is produced)
super, supra	above	+infection = superinfection (infection above or in addition to an existing one)

Suffix	Meaning	Example
-algia	pain	an (not) + algia = analgesic (something that stops pain)
-ectomy	cut out, remove surgically	appendix + ectomy = appendectomy (removal of the appendix)
-genic	origin	psyche (mind) + genic = psychogenic (originating in the mind)
-itis	inflam-mation	bursa (portion of shoulder joint) + itis = bursitis (inflammation of the bursa)
-gram	measure	electro (electric) + cardio (heart) + gram = electrocardiogram (electric measurement of heart activity)
-oma	tumor	melan (pigment) + oma = melanoma (pigmented tumor)
-osis	disease process, condition	acid + osis = disturbance in acid-base balance of body

ostomy	surgical creation of passage or opening	ilio (portion of intestine) + rect + ostomy = iliorectostomy (surgical formation of a passage between ileum and rectum)
-path -pathy	disease, pathology	idio (cause unknown) + pathic = idiopathic, pathology whose cause is unknown
-plasty	surgical shaping	naso (pertaining to the nose) + plasty = nasoplasty ("nose job")

Root	Meaning	Example
angi/o	vessel	+graph (picture) = angiograph (x-ray of a blood vessel)
arthr/o	joint	+itis (inflammation) = arthritis (inflamed joints)
bronch/i	airways to lung	+ itis = bronchitis (inflamed membranes of lung airways)
carcin/o	cancer	+genic (cause) = carcinogenic (cancer causing)
cardi/o	heart	+arrest (stoppage) = cardiac arrest (heart attack)

derm/ato	skin	+ologist (one who knows or studies) = dermatologist (skin doctor)
enter/o	intestine, bowel	+ itis (inflamed) = enteritis (irritated intestine)
gastr/o	stomach	+ulcer (sore) = gastric ulcer (sore on the stomach)
hepat/o	liver	+itis = hepatitis (inflamed, usually infected, liver)
my/o	muscle	+algia (pain) = myalgia (muscle pain)
neur/o	nerve	+plasty (surgical shaping) = neuroplasty (reconstructive surgery of a nerve)
thorac/o	chest	+centesis (puncture) = thoracocentesis (surgical puncture of the chest wall for removal of fluids)

MEDICATIONS —
THEY SHOULD HELP YOU,
NOT HURT YOU

by Robert J. Skeist, R. N.

In the United States of America

- Twenty tons of aspirin are swallowed each day.

- Fifty million prescriptions a year are written for Valium.

- One and a half million people each year are hospitalized for problems caused by medications.

- People over 65 are only 10% of the population but take 25% of the medications.

- Drug companies spend more than $4,000 per doctor each year advertising their products.

We live in a drug-happy culture. Red pills, blue pills, polka-dot pills, "nerve" pills, "water" pills, pills to wake you up, pills to put you to sleep, prescription drugs, over-the-counter drugs, the medication I just got, your medication saved from three years ago. The average visit to a doctor lasts less than 15 minutes and often focuses on medication. Many doctors ignore the importance of diet, exercise, and relaxation to their patients' health. Many people do not feel they have been helped by a doctor unless they leave the office with magic Latin words scratched onto little sheets of white paper. Any medication has the potential of causing unpleasant side effects. Many people over 65 take several different medications that may mix together and give them additional problems.

Another aspect of the medication problem is the behavior of the drug producers in our capitalist system. According to Dr. Quentin Young of Chicago's Cook County Hospital, "pharmaceuticals is one of the nation's most profitable industries, yielding profits on market investment in the range of 20%. (General Motors is happy with 1-2%.) The primary interest of these companies is not to assure our health, but to assure their profits." For constipation, loneliness or high blood pressure, drug manufacturers will not recommend better diet, friendship groups, or meditation. Nor will they even suggest purchasing the cheapest effective medication. They will urge us to buy their products. Busy doctors are bombarded with a total of $2,500,000,000 of pharmaceutical advertising annually and often rely on this information when they prescribe drugs for us. And we ourselves are affected by the barrage of medication advertisements on television and in magazines.

Older people are faced with the fact that their bodies are slowing down. Just as you do not digest a meal at age 60 as quickly as you did at age 35, your body does not use up a dose of medicine as quickly as when you were younger. While 2 mg. of a certain tranquilizer may be taken in stride by a 30-year-old, it may knock out someone 70 years old. The older person is more sensitive to the medication and more likely to suffer from side effects.

"Hey, wait a minute!" I imagine a reader objecting. "Medications have helped my mother get along with her heart condition and arthritis!" You have a good point. Correcting and strengthening a heart beat, reducing arthritis pain and swelling, bringing high blood pressure down into a safe range, fighting infections, controlling seizures, supplying insulin to diabetics — these are just a few of the valuable services drugs perform. Taken properly, drugs can prolong life or make it more pleasant. But they should not be used unnecessarily, casually, in dangerous combinations or without proper supervision, so that the "cure" becomes an additional problem.

Let's get on to some practical advice for taking medications safely.

1. *Don't take a medication unless you need it.* No medicine is candy. Any medicine has the possibility of upsetting your body. Don't demand that your doctor give you a prescription; first explore non-drug alternatives.

Never take pills from a friend because "after all, they helped me."

2. *Know the name and purpose of each medication you take.* Pity the man who confused his Doxidan with his Doriden, and took a laxative when he meant to take a sleeping pill. And what about the woman who didn't know the new pill she was taking was called dicoumarol and that it was a blood thinner? She and the Emergency Room doctor were both very surprised when a small scratch from gardening kept on bleeding. And then there is the case of the man taking a "heart pill" and a "water pill." His doctor told him to stop taking the "water pill." He figured that the "water pill" must be less important, and that the less important pill must be the smaller of the two. So he stopped taking the tiny white pill. Soon his heart beat was way off, and he wound up in the hospital. That was a hard way to learn a basic point: know the name and purpose of each medication you take.

3. *Know how to take each medication.* That may sound silly to you. After all, you just open up and swallow it down, and you can't go wrong, right? Wrong. Some antibiotics act more powerfully when taken on an empty stomach. Iron supplements, on the other hand, may be extremely irritating to an empty stomach, and

should be taken at mealtime. An "enteric-coated" pill must be swallowed whole; if you chew it, the acid in your stomach will knock out its strength. But you should chew antacid tablets until they turn to mush so that your upset stomach is spared the extra work of breaking the tablet apart. Some pills you don't swallow at all. Nitroglycerine, which is taken to relieve angina ("heart pain") must be placed under the tongue to melt. So get specific instructions for taking each of your medications.

4. *Take each medication on schedule.* One man got into trouble by skipping his blood pressure medication on days when he felt good, and taking two pills on days when he felt bad. By not following his doctor's directions to take one pill every morning, his blood pressure got out of control again.

Taking medications on schedule helps keep the right amount of medication in your blood stream at all times. Here are some suggestions that may be helpful:

- Set an alarm clock for the time to take your next medication.

- Keep a chart on your refrigerator or medicine cabinet listing when you should take each dose.

- If you really have trouble remembering when to take your medications, have a friend, relative, or home health aide call in the morning to remind you or come by to set out your whole day's medications for you in labelled containers.

Instructions may be provided on your medication labels using these or other abbreviations:

a.c.	before meals
ad lib	freely, as desired
b.i.d.	two times a day
c̄	with
caps.	capsule
gtt	a drop
hr	hour
h.s.	hour of sleep, bedtime
i	one
ii	two
o.d.	every day
O. D.	right eye
o.h.	every hour
o.n.	every night
O. S.	left eye
os	mouth
p.c.	after meals
PO	by mouth
PR	by rectum
PRN	when required
q̄	every
q.d.	every day
q.h.	every hour
q.i.d.	four times a day
q.o.d.	every other day
s̄	without
ss	one half
tab.	tablet
t.i.d.	three times a day
ung.	ointment

5. *Ask your doctor if your drugs will cause problems if you take them with other medications, alcohol, or food.*

For example, if antacids are taken at the same time as the antibiotic tetracycline, the tetracycline loses its effectiveness. Aspirin should not be taken along with Motrin, Indocin, or other prescription arthritis medication. If taken together, neither the aspirin nor the prescription medications will work as well. Aspirin may also cause problems for someone taking a "blood thinner" (anti-coagulant). Together they may thin the blood so much that the person bleeds too easily.

If you have an alcoholic drink or two along with a sleeping pill, a Valium, or anything else you use to calm you down, you may wind up dangerously "tranquil." Alcohol and tranquilizers taken together produce an "additive effect — each one makes the other work more strongly than usual. Also, alcohol consumed with antidiabetic agents may lead to a dangerously lowered blood sugar level.

Drug/food interactions are another consideration. The antibiotic tetracycline will not work properly if taken with milk or any dairy product. Calcium in these products attaches to the medication and makes it useless. Another example relates to the anti-depressants known as MAO-inhibitors, which are dangerous in combination with certain cheeses, chocolate, beverages, and other foods.

6. *Be alert for side effects.*

Mr. Jones has a headache and takes two aspirin. His headache goes away, but he gets an upset stomach.

Mr. Anderson, age 67, starts taking a new medication for his blood pressure. Four months later, his blood pressure isn't the only thing that is down. Troubled for the first time by impotence (unable to have an erection), he figures he is "just too old for sex." He also develops a stuffy nose, and treats it with an over-the-counter cold medication that slightly raises his blood pressure.

For the past three years, Mrs. Levine has been taking a "water pill" (diuretic). She now develops nausea and muscle cramps, caused by passing too much potassium in her urine.

Mrs. Smith starts on a new blood pressure medication. Several months later she is very depressed, forgetful, and short-tempered. Her son decides she is getting senile, and starts to consider placing her in a nursing home.

Mr. Jackson had been taking a "blood thinner" (anti-coagulant) ever since his heart attack six months ago. He has frequent headaches and takes several aspirin tablets a day. One afternoon he is gardening, gets a small scratch, and bleeds so much that he has to go to the Emergency Room.

What do these five people have in common? They are suffering from side effects of medications. Drugs they take to cope with medical problems have caused upset stomach, impotence, nausea, cramping, confusion, and bleeding. Other possible side effects from various medications include dizziness, diarrhea, anxiety, ringing in the ears, and rashes.

It is a good idea to ask your doctor and pharmacist about what side effects to watch out for and how you might avoid them. Let's take a fresh look at our five friends who learned about side effects the hard way.

Mr. Jones could have avoided his upset stomach by taking acetaminophen (sold as a generic product or as Tylenol or Datril), or by crushing his aspirin and taking it with a little food.

If Mr. Anderson had told his doctor that he had developed sexual problems, his doctor may have been able to improve the situation by decreasing the dose or changing medications. If he had mentioned his stuffed nose, his doctor would have had a chance to warn against the use of preparations that raise the blood pressure.

Orange juice or a banana each morning with breakfast might have provided Mrs. Levine with enough potassium to make up for what she lost in her urine. Or she might take a potassium supplement provided by her doctor.

Mrs. Smith may wind up in a nursing home. It could be her medication that is affecting her mood and her memory. That side effect, combined with the common stereotype that "old people are senile," makes for plenty of trouble. Let's hope that before she — or anyone — is sent off to a nursing home, a thorough medication check is done.

And what Mr. Jackson needed was some simple advice — to use very little aspirin while on a "blood thinner," and to have his blood clotting time checked periodically.

By now you will understand this advice: First, ask your doctor and your pharmacist what side effects might come from your medications and what you can do about them. Second, if you are taking any medications and develop any physical or emotional problems, insist that your doctor and pharmacist review all of your medications. If you feel that one of your medications is upsetting you, don't just decide to stop taking it. Please, call your doctor and talk it over. Perhaps what you are feeling is *not* a side effect from your medication, and stopping the medication would create additional problems. Or perhaps you are experiencing a side effect, but what you need is a smaller dose or a different medication, rather than no medication at all.

7. *Store your medications safely.*

How you store your medications may affect how long they "keep." Often the label has instructions, such as "store in a cool, dry place." Unless specifically labelled "refrigerate," medications should not be stored in refrigerators, since the humidity there may break them down.

If is best to keep each medication in a separate container. Mixed together, the chemicals of one pill may change another pill. Another safety rule is, don't switch medications that come in dark containers into clear containers. They may be sensitive to light. Nitroglycerine is an example — it goes "bad" very quickly if light gets at it.

If I ever go to work as a tour guide of historical Chicago sites, there are a few medication cabinets I'd like to include. They contain bottles of pills and potions from 10, 20, 30, or 40 years ago. This is good history, but bad medicine. Lots of medications change over the years. They could be stronger, weaker, or just different than they are supposed to be.

Once a year, give your medication cabinet a good cleaning. Get rid of anything over two years old. Some medicines, like Nitroglycerine, last only a few months before they should be thrown out.

8. *Go easy with over-the-counter medications.*

Anyone can walk into a drug store and buy all sorts of drugs without any prescription. This does not mean they are harmless.

- If you're using any non-prescription medication for more than a week, tell your doctor. It may be a clue to a problem that needs treatment.

- If you need to avoid sodium, caffeine, or other substances, check the labels. "Alka-Seltzer," for example, contains caffeine and sodium.

- Laxatives can be habit-forming. It is better to regulate bowel movements through diet and exercise.

- Certain fat-soluble vitamins (A, D, E) may be harmful in large quantities. (But a daily multi-vitamin is safe.)

9. *Ask for your prescription to be written for and filled with a low-cost generic product.*

Pharmacies often carry the same medication from several different companies. For example, let's talk about a common "water pill" or diuretic, hydrochlorothiazide. This is the *generic name*, which no one can patent. Eighteen companies make hydrochlorothiazide and sell it by that name. Three other companies make the hydrochlorothiazide but use their own *brand names*: CIBA calls it Esidrex; Merck Sharp & Dohme calls it Hydrodiuril; and Abbott calls it Oretic. A brand name may be used by only one company.

According to the Food and Drug Administration, all 21 of these drugs have been shown to work the same way. The big difference is in the price tag. At my neighborhood pharmacy, the generic form of this water pill goes for half the price of the brand name. Why pay twice as much for a catchy name?

So ask your pharmacist if there is a generic drug that may be used to fill your prescription. If you send someone to the drug store to pick up your medication, give this person a signed note saying, "I authorize _____ to pick up my medication in a lower-cost generic equivalent."

It is occasionally a good idea not to substitute. Perhaps you are delicately balanced on a certain medication, and your doctor does not want to risk the slightest variation. Sometimes the way a medicine is colored or held together makes it work a little differently than another company's version of the same medicine. Very rarely, a doctor has reliable information (i.e., provided by an objective scientific source and not by the companies that make the drugs and have a financial incentive to distort the truth) that one company puts out a better quality medication than any other company. Sometimes it is impossible to substitute a generic product, since the original developer of a medication maintains exclusive control of the formula for 17 years.

Through careful shopping you can cut down further on your medication costs. Some drugs store very well and can be purchased at a discount in large quantities. The American Association of Retired Persons (1909 K Street, N. W., Washington, D. C. 20034) offers a reputable mail-order service.

10. *Keep a record of your medications.* It is important to have in your wallet a list of all of your prescription and over-the-counter drugs. This is useful to you for remembering your doctors' and pharmacists' instructions, and to medical personnel for understanding your situation better in an emergency. Below is a sample of a card that folds to wallet size. Thousands of these have been distributed through the Seniors' Health Program of Augustana Hospital in Chicago.

Robert J. Skeist

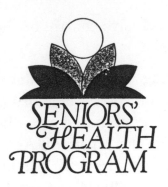

Augusīana

HOSPITAL AND
HEALTH CARE CENTER

411 WEST DICKENS AVENUE
CHICAGO, ILLINOIS 60614
312 975 5056

MY MEDICATIONS

PERSONAL INFORMATION

Name

Address   City

Date of Birth   Phone

Contact in Emergency   Phone

Ins. No.

Medical Conditions

Doctor

Doctor

Pharmacist

Other

MEDICATION (Prescription & Over-the-Counter)	FOR WHAT CONDITION	DOSAGE	WHEN AND HOW TO TAKE
1.	1.	1.	1.
2.	2.	2.	2.
3.	3.	3.	3.
4.	4.	4.	4.
5.	5.	5.	5.
6.	6.	6.	6.
7.	7.	7.	7.
8.	8.	8.	8.

A final reminder: Ask questions. It is my job as a nurse, and the job of your own doctors, nurses, and pharmacists, to give you the information you need to understand whether to take a medication and how to take it so it helps you.

For further reading:

The Elderly: Their Health and the Drugs in their Lives, by Michael J. Gaeta, M. S. Ed. and Ronald J. Gaetano R. Ph. 1977; 122 pages $6.45 from Kendall/Hall Publishing Company, Dubuque, Iowa 52001. A large-type, highly-readable, consumer-oriented book providing information and precautions related to medications for high blood pressure, cancer, diabetes, and other diseases as well as caffeine, alcohol, and tobacco.

Handbook of Non-Prescription Drugs, Cynthia Kleinfield, Editor 1979; 512 pages $20.00 postpaid from the American Pharmaceutical Association, 2215 Constitution Avenue, N. W., Washington, D. C. 20037. Discusses in plain English thousands of over-the-counter products including pain relievers, antacids, laxatives.

The People's Pharmacy by Joe Graedon 1976; 401 pages. $4.95 postpaid from Avon Books, 959 Eighth Avenue, New York, N. Y. 10019. Written by a pharmacologist for the general public, it provides guidance on prescription drugs plus "money-saving home remedies."

The Pill Book by Harold M. Silverman. Pharm. D. , and Gilbert I. Simon, D. Sc. 1979; 417 pages. $3.70 postpaid from Bantam Books, 414 East Golf Road, Des Plaines, Illinois 60016. A handy book for the lay person to check on over 900 prescription drugs for general information, possible side effects, usual dose, and more.

For wallet-sized medication safety cards, samples of consumer-education fliers and other information related to drug education with older people, write to *Seniors' Health Program*, Augustana Hospital, 411 W. Dickens, Chicago, Illinois 60614.

PAYING THE BILLS: A Guide to Medicare, Supplemental Insurance, and Medicaid

by J. Ram Ray

The Medicare program held a tremendous promise for meeting the health care needs of the elderly when it was first enacted in 1965. Unfortunately, we have not seen the fulfillment of that promise.

U. S. House Select Committee on Aging

Everyone is talking about the crisis in health care, whopping hospital bills, and the need for national health insurance. But the debate over national health insurance makes no reference to the special health needs of persons 65 or older. Everyone seems to think that grandpa and grandma are protected by Medicare and have nothing to worry about.

In fact, nothing can be farther from reality. Medicare, the Federal Government's medical insurance program for people over 65, covers only a part of the medical expenses of the elderly, and this part keeps decreasing every year. What Medicare does not cover plays havoc with the pocket-books of elderly people on fixed incomes.

There will be more and more old people in the years to come, because people are living longer. So, our society will have to provide health care to growing numbers of elderly. If our present system of health care does not change, we are in for serious trouble.

Before we talk about why Medicare is not enough, let us talk a little about what it is, what it covers, and how much it costs.

Medicare at a Glance

"The elderly are sick more frequently and for more prolonged periods than the rest of the population. For every 100 persons age 65 and over, 80 suffer some kind of chronic ailment. Sixteen are hospitalized one or more times annually."

President Kennedy sent this message to the Congress in February 1963, urging the enactment of Medicare, a program that became law in 1965. Congress did not intend it as a total health care package, but as a hedge against major sickness wiping out a retired person's life savings in one stroke. In the beginning at least, Medicare did a good job of meeting this need.

Medicare has two parts: Part A, hospital insurance; and Part B, medical insurance. If you are on

Social Security, you are automatically eligible for Part A. For Part B, you pay a monthly premium. This premium has been increasing with inflation, and, as of December 1978, is $8.20 a month.

Information on what Medicare does and does not cover is written in insurance jargon. Here are the most frequently-used terms and what they mean:

Deductible — If you own a car, you know how auto insurance works: you pay the first $100.00, $150.00, or $200.00 of the repair costs every time you make a claim on your policy. Medicare deductible is the amount you have to pay before the insurance steps in.

Co-payment — This is the percentage of your hospital or medical bills that you must pay. For example, if surgery costs $600.00 and Medicare pays 80%, your co-payment is 20% of $600.00, or $120.00

Reasonable fees or allowable charges — Medicare pays for hospital and doctor services according to a schedule it follows, depending on what it considers to be "reasonable" costs in your area. This is one of the major pitfalls of Medicare, as we shall see later.

Pre-existing condition — Health problems you have or have had in the past are often not covered at all, or not covered for a period of time specified in the policy. You will run into pre-existing condition clauses a lot when dealing with Medicare supplement policies, discussed later in this chapter. For example, if you have had a heart attack, your policy may not cover heart attacks during the first six months of your policy or may not cover them at all.

Benefit period — All Medicare benefits are provided per benefit period. A benefit period starts the day you enter hospital or nursing home and continues for up to 60 days. You must be in a hospital or nursing home for a total of 60 days before the next period starts. For example, if you break your leg and spend 10 days in a hospital, then re-enter hospital after a month for a gall bladder operation, your benefit period will continue with day 11.

What Medicare Covers

The following table shows what Medicare pays and what you pay, as of December 1978:

Medicare Pays	You Pay
PART A (Hospital insurance)	
Complete inpatient services for the first 60 days	$144.00 deductible
Inpatient services 61st to 90th day	$31.00 per day
Lifetime reserve of 60 additional days	$62.00 per day
Nursing care for the first 20 days in a nursing home, after a minimum of 3 days in a hospital	Nothing
Nursing home care 21st to 100th day	$18.00 per day from 21st to 100th day, and full charges for anything over 100 days.

Medicare Pays	You Pay
PART B (Medical insurance) 80% of "reasonable fee" for doctor visits, outpatient services, and surgery	$60.00 deductible, plus 20% of all doctor charges, outpatient services, and surgery. AND any amount over what Medicare considers "reasonable."

This table is by no means complete. Medicare also pays for 80% of doctors' charges while you are in a nursing home, for limited home health care equipment, and fir visits by nurses and physical therapists. These and other benefits are explained in detail in *Your Medicare Handbook,* available free from any local Social Security Office.

What Medicare does NOT Cover

"Medicare was set up by people who knew nothing about aging."

Dr. Robert Butler, Director
National Institute on Aging

The basic pitfall of Medicare is that it was designed to cover medical bills and not health care services. It does not pay for medical check-ups, medications, eye glasses, flu shots, dental care, dentures, hearing aids, visits to the foot doctor, and other day-to-day health needs.

Granting that Medicare covers only serious illness and not routine health care, it does a poor job of even that. Medicare will not pay for a private room in a hospital, unless your doctor says you absolutely need it. It will not pay for a private nurse. It will not pay for your use of a telephone or television set while you are in hospital. If you need blood, Medicare will not pay for the first three pints.

Medicare may refuse to pay for certain tests and hospital services, if it feels they are not necessary in your case. Your doctor may disagree with Medicare, but that will not make any difference.

"All right," you may say. "After all, Medicare is not total insurance, and will not pay for everything. I can live with that." But the problems do not end there. Medicare may not fully cover even those bills it said it would pay. It pays only what it considers "reasonable" for surgery and other doctor services.

Suppose you need gall bladder surgery, for which your surgeon charges $750.00. Medicare's "reasonable" fee for this operation may be only $600.00, in which case it would pay only 80% of $600.00, or $480.00. The other $270.00 would come out of your pocket.

Because of the "reasonable fee" provision and the difficulty many have in paying the remainder of their bills, some doctors discourage Medicare patients from coming to them or actually refuse to treat them. Even officials in the Social Security Administration, which runs Medicare, admit that the "reasonable fee" schedule is often outdated and based on fees prevailing two or three years earlier.

In 1975, Medicare ruled that 75% of the doctors' bills submitted to them reflected "unreasonable fees." Medicare cut these bills an average of 17% — up from 14% in 1974 — before paying its share. In the Chicago area between January and June 1978, Medicare cited the same provision to reduce or reject a whopping 84% of claims processed. There is widespread sentiment that physicians' fees and incomes in this country are beyond what is reasonable. It is ironic and unjust that older people on fixed incomes should be penalized for this.

Often, people do not even get the coverage they are legally entitled to. Congress' General Accounting Office recently conducted a spot check of Medicare claims processed by Blue Cross/Blue Shield in

New York and found incorrect or unfair reductions in 13% of the cases.

How do these statistics translate into dollars and cents for the person over 65? According to the highly respected *Consumer Reports* magazine (January 1976) the average Medicare patient in 1975 spent $1,218.00 on medical care. Of this, Medicare covered only $463.00.

Supplements to Medicare Insurance

As Medicare's coverage became worse year after year, private insurance companies stepped in with their wares. Often referred to as "Medi-gap insurance" or "Medicare wrap-around," supplement to Medicare insurance is now one of the fastest-growing segments of the insurance industry. Nearly half of all Medicare participants also carry Medicare supplement insurance. Insurance executives say this is a $1 billion-a-year market! Several national and local companies sell Medicare supplement policies. They are not all alike. Some companies offer a basic policy to cover Medicare deductibles, with additional coverage optional at extra premium. Others offer various policies to pay for items not covered by Medicare. *No Medicare supplement policy covers all the gaps left by Medicare.* It is not possible here to examine each of the hundreds of policies on the market, but the following table (based on information available in December 1978) will help you choose the supplemental policy that offers the best coverage for your money:

Part A

1. Maximum Benefit Payable
2. Deductible for the First 60 Days ($160.00).
3. Deductible From 61st Through 90th Day ($40.00 Per Day).
4. Lifetime Deductible ($80.00 Per Day) For 60 Days Lifetime Reserve.
5. Hospital Benefits Payable After Expiration of Lifetime Reserve.
6. Deductible of $20.00 Per Day for Skilled Nursing Home Care. 21st — 100 Day.
7. Are Nursing Home Benefits Paid After 100 Days?
8. For Payment of Benefits in a Skilled Nursing Home Care Center, is Medicare Approval and/or Medicare Payment Necessary?
9. Blanket Policy or Different Policies?

	Intercontinental Life Insurance Co.	Mutual of Omaha	National Council of Senior Citizens
1.	None	$10,000	No Limit
2.	Covered	Covered	No
3.	Covered	Covered	Covered
4.	Covered	Covered	Covered
5.	None	Yes	Yes
6.	Covered	Covered	Covered
7.	No	Yes	Yes
8.	Yes	Yes	Yes
9.	Nursing Home Care Optional	Blanket	Blanket

	AARP Mature Care — 65 (Colonial Penn)	Blue Shield/ Blue Cross 65 (Chicago)	Illinois Assn. of Senior Citizens Pioneer Life of Illinois
1.	$50,000	820 Days	No Limit
2.	Covered	Covered	Covered
3.	Covered	Covered	Covered
4.	Covered	Covered	Covered
5.	$75 Per Day	670 Days	$72 Per Day
6.	Covered	Covered	Covered
7.	$13.50 Per Day	No	No
8.	Yes	Yes	No
9.	Blanket	Blanket	Blanket

	National Old Line Insurance Co.	Reliable Life and Casualty Co.	Union Fidelity
1.	No Limit	$25,000	$50,000
2.	Covered	Covered	Covered
3.	Covered	Covered	Covered
4.	Covered	Covered	Covered
5.	$100 Per Day	$40 Per Day	$50,000 Limit
6.	Covered	Covered	Covered
7.	Yes	No	No
8.	Yes	No	Yes
9.	Nursing Home Care Optional	Optional Riders At Extra Cost	Blanket

Part B

1. Maximum Benefit Payable —
2. Are Medical/Surgical Expense Benefits Payable if Medicare Disallows Charges or Does Not Authorize Coverages.
3. Initial Deductible for Doctor Charges ($60.00) Per Calendar Year.
4. 20% Deductible of Medical/Surgical Charges.
5. 20% Deductible for Out-Patient Services Including Surgical.
6. 20% of Doctor Visits while in a Nursing Home.

General Provisions

7. Waiting Period For New Conditions.
8. Waiting Period For Pre-Existing Health Conditions.
9. Maximum Age of Issue.
10. Is Policy Issued Without Restrictive Endorsements or Riders?
11. Is Policy Contract Guaranteed Renewable?

	Intercontinental Life Insurance Co.	Mutual of Omaha	National Council of Senior Citizens
1.	$1,000	$5,000	No Limit
2.	No	No	No
3.	Yes	Yes	No
4.	Covered	Covered	Covered
5.	No	Covered	Covered
6.	No	Yes	Yes
7.	None	None	None
8.	6 Months	6 Months	6 Months
9.	None	None	None
10.	Specified	Yes	Yes
11.	Yes	Yes	Yes

	AARP Mature Care — 65 (Colonial Penn)	Blue Shield/ Blue Cross 65 (Chicago)	Illinois Assn. of Senior Citizens Pioneer Life of Illinois
1.	$50,000	None	No Limit
2.	No	No	Yes
3.	20% of in patient expenses only	20% only	Yes
4.	Covered	Covered	Covered
5.	Covered	Covered	Covered
6.	Covered	Covered	Covered
7.	None	None	None
8.	3 Months	None	3 Months
9.	None	None	None
10.	Yes	Yes	Yes
11.	Yes	No	Yes

	National Old Line Insurance Co.	Reliable Life and Casualty Co.	Union Fidelity
1.	No Limit	$400	20% of Doctor and Surgery Charges Only
2.	No	Yes	No
3.	Yes	Yes	No
4.	Covered	Covered	Covered
5.	Covered	Covered	No
6.	No	No	No
7.	None	None	Not Available
8.	5 Months	3 Months	Not Available
9.	None	None	None
10.	Yes	Yes	Yes
11.	Yes	Yes	No

When choosing an insurance company, I recommend these guidelines:

- A good Medicare supplement policy should cover as many Medicare gaps as possible. You can reject the policy outright if it does not cover the basic deductibles shown in the chart on page 000.

- Look for policies that cover the basic deductibles and offer additional coverage — for private hospital rooms, private nurses, doctors' fees for outpatient visits and house calls, etc. at extra premium. Such policies are superior to those which offer only partial coverage, which means you have to buy different policies to obtain complete coverage.

- Policies that offer "service" benefits (a percentage of actual charges) are superior to those that offer "indemnity" benefits (a fixed amount for each service or each day in hospital).

- No time limit, or a short time limit, for pre-existing conditions is another point to look for. Most policies have clauses for pre-existing conditions from three months to one year; reject any policy with a limit of more than six months.

- Most Medicare supplement policies on the market pay benefits based on Medicare's notion of "reasonable fees." Going back to our earlier example, if a surgeon charges you $750.00 for gall bladder surgery and Medicare says the "reasonable fee" for the surgery is only $600.00, most insurance policies cover 20% of the $600.00 and don't help you at all with the remaining $150. A few policies have a provision to pay benefits for doctors' charges beyond what Medicare considers "reasonable." It is preferable to choose one of these policies, if offered by a reputable company. I stress the word "reputable" because any insurance policy, no matter what it states, is only as good as the company backing it.

Remember, insurance companies are in the business for profits — not out of concern for your health. Insurance companies practically invented the *fine print;* it may take a lawyer to understand the language contained in insurance policies. What you read in the sales brochure may not be exactly what you get in the policy.

Every insurance company doing business in your state is required to register with the State Department (or Commission) of Insurance, and obtain a license to sell insurance in the state. Every insurance agent is also required to pass an examination and obtain a license.

You can call your State Department of Insurance to find out if an insurance company or agent is licensed in your state and to get a full explanation of policy terms that confuse you. You can also request a social worker in the senior center in your neighborhood to check on an insurance company. Or, you can call the local Better Business Bureau for this information.

State insurance departments are frequently accused of protecting the insurance interests instead of consumers — an accusation not entirely unfair. Recently, the Legal Aid Bureau in Rockford, Illinois filed a complaint with the Illinois Department of Insurance about an insurance salesman, after he had duped several old women living alone. The Insurance Department did not respond to the complaint and, when contacted about the matter several weeks later by a newspaper reporter, said it did not see sufficient reason to cancel the salesman's license.

Insurance agents specializing in Medicare supplement insurance are known for preying on elderly persons, especially women living alone. My advice here is, never buy from a door-to-door salesman. Period! If a salesman knocks at your door, tell him (without opening your door) to leave his sales brochures at the door and leave, and you will write to the company if you decide to buy. Never let a salesman talk you into buying a policy you don't need. Never listen to a salesman who tells you that your present policy is no good and you should cancel it.

Remember, each new policy has a pre-existing condition provision, and you may be sacrificing important protection when you switch.

Many agents who represent several companies try to sell the same person two or more policies, often with duplicate coverages. Remember, no matter how many policies you have, you can collect for a given item from only one policy.

Never buy an insurance policy simply because it is endorsed by a club or association you belong to, such as the American Association of Retired Persons (which is connected to Colonial Penn organizationally and financially) or the National Council of Senior Citizens. If the policy does not meet the standards described earlier, don't buy it.

If you do not understand the fine print on your policy, ask a worker at the local senior center to help you. If you buy a policy and then have second thoughts, you can return it to the insurance company within 10 days after you buy it and get a full refund; some companies allow up to one month for cancellation with full refund.

Despite their limitations, Medicare supplement insurance policies fill a real need. A good policy can save you the basic deductibles each benefit period, and most policies cost you less than the basic combined deductibles ($144.00 under Part A and $60.00 under Part B). For example, Blue Cross/Blue Shield-65 offered by the Blue Cross of Chicago costs less than $120.00 a year and covers the basic deductibles. Some policies pay for hospital stay beyond the 90 days covered by Medicare, so you don't have to use up your 60 Lifetime Reserve Days. A Medicare supplement policy that covers prolonged stay in a nursing home can save you a bundle. Remember, after you finish 100 days in a nursing home, Medicare leaves you on your own. You will be eligible for Medicaid, the government program for health care for the poor, but not before you spend all your liquid assets, such as savings, stocks, and other holdings.

If you are 70 years or over, or if you have a chronic ailment, such as a heart condition or diabetes, then you should buy a long-term care policy to supplement your Medicare.

Medicaid

Medicaid is not the same as Medicare. Medicaid is the Federal Government's health care program for the poor, administered by state governments. If your income is less than $180.00 a month ($227.00 per couple) and you are not covered by Medicare, you are eligible for Medicaid, which pays for all hospital and medical care. However, even if your income is low, if you have more than a very small amount of assets, then you are not eligible for Medicaid. In Illinois, for example, you can own a house for your use, a car, a savings account of no more than $400.00, and life insurance of no more than $1,000.00, and still be eligible for Medicaid. But if you own a house and you get on Medicaid, then a lien will be placed against your house. That is, when you or your heirs sell the house, the government will collect what it paid for your health care.

If you are on Medicare but your income is less than $180.00 a month ($227.00 per couple) and you own no property other than a house, a car, and savings of less than $400.00, then Medicaid will pay for those parts of your hospital and medical bills not covered by Medicare. A social worker in the hospital will take care of this for you.

Fighting Back

When Medicare rejects or reduces your claims, you can appeal to your local Social Security Office for reconsideration. A social worker at the local senior center can help you prepare your appeal. If your claims are not settled to your satisfaction, write to your Congressman or your Senator. Medicare claims promptly settled after telephone calls from Congressmen's or Senators' offices are not uncommon.

If you think a Medicare supplement policy does not serve the needs of those it is intended for, you can write to your State Department of Insurance and try to get the policy changed. Recently, Ed Grant, a 77-year-old retired advertising salesman, saw a new rider on the Blue Cross policies which gave the insurance company and not the doctor last say in deciding what medical services are necessary. Mr. Grant brought the matter to the attention of the Director of the Illinois Department of Insurance, who wrote to Blue Cross, officially disapproving the new rider. Thanks to Ed Grant's initiative, Blue Cross was forced to withdraw the rider.

The Federal government paid more than $22 billion in Medicare benefits in 1977 and about $25 billion in 1978. The government is under pressure from labor and senior citizen groups to expand Medicare coverage. But the chances of Medicare paying for eye glasses, prescription drugs, and other items are remote. These would add an additional $15 billion to Medicare, clearly out of the question in the post-Proposition 13 politics.

Medicare, Medicaid, and Medi-gap insurance policies together do not present a comprehensive health care plan for the elderly. They are like a number of Band-Aids where major surgery is needed. In the short run, we need Medicare revisions that provide for coverage of more medical expenses for the nation's elderly. In the long run, we not only need a new system to pay our medical bills, but also a new approach — one that de-emphasizes medical solutions to health problems and stresses health education, early detection of problems, regular exercise, safe working conditions, a cleaner environment, and the availability of good food and housing for all of our people.

HOW THINGS SHOULD BE

CHANGING THE MEDICAL SYSTEM:
AN INTERVIEW
WITH ROBERT N. BUTLER, M. D.
by Robert J. Skeist, R.N.

Dr. Butler received his medical degree from the Columbia University College of Physicians and Surgeons. He is the first Director of the National Institute on Aging of the National Institute of Health, a federal agency whose purpose is to support and conduct biomedical and behavioral research in aging to enhance the quality of later life. He was formerly on the faculties of the Howard University and George Washington University Schools of Medicine, the Washington School of Psychiatry, and Washington Psychoanalytic Institute. He is the author of Why Survive? Being Old in America *and co-author with* Myrna Lewis *of* Love and Sex After Sixty. *What follows is an edited version of my conversation with Dr. Butler in 1979.*

RS: *What changes in health care for older people do you hope to see in the next 20 years?*

RB: We are now witnessing one of those necessary changes, a rapid increase in geriatric medical education. For example, I just met with the Board of Internists. They have decided that their exam for certification will include information related to aging. Now it's just a matter of formulating the questions. The point is that new doctors are expected to understand the aging process. The medical schools and schools of osteopathy have responded to our suggestions and our urging much more quickly than I had ever hoped.

Part of my discussion with all the medical schools is that the issue is not only content but attitude. Medical students refer to elderly patients with terms such as "crock" and "old biddy" out of their own nervousness about aging. A lot of them have no contact with or understanding of healthy old people. They think "old" equals "sick". That leads us to another pressing need — the creation of health promotion and disease prevention clinics for the elderly.

RS: *I work at a health promotion program at Augustana Hospital in Chicago. One of our main concerns is the misuse and overuse of medications. Do you think there really is a drug problem for older people?*

RB: Yes, and for those of us who work with the elderly. There is a lot of overprescription by doctors in the community and in nursing homes, without due attention to alternatives or to the kind of interactions that can occur. There's not much change yet, and not only because of doctors. We have a huge pharmaceutical industry that keeps pushing for the increased use of medications.

RS: *At Cook County Hospital in Chicago, due in part to the efforts of Dr. Quentin Young, head of the Department of Medicine, they're addressing the medication issue on an institutional level. They have banned detail men (drug company salesmen) from the hospital, cut down on the use of tranquilizers by increasing doctor-patient contact, and decided to use mostly generic drugs.*

RB: That sounds like the way to be moving. I'd like more information on that so I can tell other people, "Look how they're facing the medication issue at Cook County Hospital."

RS: *Are changes in exercise and nutrition of any use to people who are already 50, 60, or 70 years old?*

RB: Of course, at any age! We have to begin with proper medical evaluation. I realize that is hard for a lot of people since Medicare doesn't provide for checkups. Then there has to be a gradual evolution — you can't jump right into a strenous program. We need a clear notion of the proper exercises for someone with arthritis, congestive heart failure, a history of heart attack, or depression.

In nursing homes, the vast majority of patients should go through exercises. This would decrease the use of medications, reduce tension, and give them a little more pleasure in life.

Now, nutrition. Here at the National Institute of Aging we're doing some studies, but we don't have the scientific base to make the proper recommendations. Still we can make a few suggestions. We've got 295,000 hip fractures in the U. S. each year; the highest risk group is older women, especially white women after the menopause. They develop osteoporosis, weak bones, as calcium leaves their bones. I think it makes sense to drink two to three glasses of skim milk each day or take a 1 gram calcium tablet.

You know we need vitamin D to make use of calcium. Anyone not out in the sunlight for a little while each day should take some vitamin D, which is usually added to milk.

People should be careful taking mineral oil laxatives, which can rob the body of fat-soluble viatmins.

For basic dietary guidelines I'm pretty much in agreement with the "McGovern Report" —

more complex carbohydrates such as whole grains, controlled amount of animal fat, plenty of fresh fruits and vegetables, less sugar, less salt.

RS: *Dr. Butler, do we need a National Health Service?*

RB: Neither the Kennedy bill nor the Carter bill for expanded insurance coverage speaks to a lot of key issues. They don't provide for improved long-term care, home care, increased reimbursement for treating old people, health promotion, or the education of doctors and nurses sensitive to the lives and needs of old people. We need a much more comprehensive national health program. An increased emphasis on occupational health is necessary, because many of our health problems are caused by day-to-day exposure to health hazards on the job.

Beyond changes in health care, we need to humanize our culture to be more sensitive to older people, to all the people who are in the shadows.

For readings on related topics:

Why Survive? Being Old in America by Robert N. Butler, M. D. , Harper and Row, 1975, New York, N. Y. $5.95. The Pulitzer Prize-winning exposé of the poor treatment of older people in our society. A call to action for all segments of our society to create the opportunity for all of us to make our lives works of art.

A Healthy State: An International Perspective on the Crisis in the United States Medical Care by Victor W. Sidel and Ruth Sidel. Pantheon Books, New York. $10.95. A physician and social worker, both leaders in the public health field, discuss health care and medical care in Sweden, Great Britain, the Soviet Union and the People's Republic of China and propose sweeping reforms of the U. S. medical system in the context of basic social and economic change.

For referral to physicians specializing in the care of older people, contact:

American Geriatrics Society
10 Columbus Circle
New York, N. Y. 10019

For additional literature, and information on the activities of the agency Dr. Butler directs, contact:

Office of Information
National Institute on Aging
Bethesda, Maryland 20014

BUILDING SUPPORT
GROUPS: Sage
and the Association for Humanistic
Gerontology
by Ken Dychtwald, Ph. D.

For the past six years, the staff and clientele of the Sage Project in Berkeley, California have been generating positive images of aging by demonstrating that people over sixty can grow and transcend the negative expectations of our culture. Through the creation of a humanistically focused self-development program for men and women over sixty years of age, they have been exploring the many ways in which the later years of life can be a time for health, vitality, expanded awareness, and the realization of self that comes from having lived a long and full life.

The Sage approach to personal growth with older adults is eclectic in technique, drawing from a wide range of Western therapeutic and self-awareness methods such as biofeedback, relaxation training, sensory awareness, gestalt, encounter, psychodrama, art and music therapy, massage, and journal writing, as well as a variety of Eastern self-developmental disciplines and processes such as meditation, yoga, tai chi, kum nye, chanting, and pranayama breathing exercises. In addition, the Sage approach to group work and individual counseling is holistic in practice, since it focuses on the individual as a whole person, working simultaneously with the mind, body, and spirit.

Sage was formed in early 1974 by Gay Luce, Eugenia Gerrard, and Ken Dychtwald. At present, the Sage staff is composed of twenty psychologists, physicians, breathing, movement, and art therapists, and specialists with extensive training in a wide variety of human arts. The Sage Project is unique in that it is the first highly successful program to merge effectively a humanistic clinical approach to self-development and personal growth with a much needed demand for creative and positively oriented gerontological programs and services.

In many instances, the Sage program has been successful in increasing the physical health, emotional stability, and self-esteem of elders.

According to Sage participant 75-year-old Herb Pillars:

> I came here afraid of dying and even more afraid of being a burden in my old age. Now I'm not nearly so afraid. . . .As for the changes, I came here with arthritis in my hands, terrible backaches, and a stiff neck. I still have a little

trouble with the arthritis, but the backache is gone, and I can now twist my head and see the traffic behind me on the road when I'm driving. Also, I used to smoke. You can't smoke and deep breathe at the same time!

Another Sage member, Ellie Karbach, 73, described herself as "an old post-cancer case with high blood pressure." Says Ellie:

At Sage I have been learning how to be alive and vital again. For example, I was recently at a party and ate some of the wrong things. When I went home, I suffered from a tachycardia (rapid heartbeat) attack. I immediately put myself into a state of deep relaxation and practiced yogic breathing, and the attack quickly passed. . . .In addition to becoming more aware of myself in a physical way, I have also been learning quite a bit about my mind and my feelings. In my Sage group I had a chance to work through some of my long-repressed grief about losing six people including my brother within a short period of time. One day I was doing my deep breathing exercises when emotions started coming up and I began to cry. . . .I wept bitterly for two hours, and I wept away a score of sorrows. And, finally, I started to laugh, thinking of all the people who have loved me all my life and still love me. . . .I'll never be the same. No one ever had a chance at age 73 to live a new life as I have.

According to Frances Burch, 68:

> I've seen people in this group change their physical and mental outlook. They're more open and responsive, their lives are more exciting, and they have more possibilities and choices. I feel much better myself. I've seen things go on here that are amazing. . . .self-healing. Here we're learning to tap new personal power sources through our spiritual growth. I'm finding energy that I haven't had in years.

At present, the Sage project has four primary programs: (a) Core group programs; (b) Institutional programs; (c) Professional training and research; and (d) National development and national networking.

The Sage core group program was the first of the various Sage experiments to gain national recognition for the way in which it was able to revitalize the minds, bodies, and spirits of its older participants. Sage core groups begin each fall and meet weekly for three, six or nine months at Sage headquarters in Berkeley, California. Composed of about twelve relatively healthy older people and two staff members, each core group becomes the medium in which staff and participants share their skills and themselves as a means of personal exploration focusing on improving physical and psychological functioning.

Graduates of Sage core groups are welcome to join the Sage core groups are welcome to join the Sage elder community, which is an action-oriented, ongoing self-help group run and coordinated entirely by core group members. In addition, core group graduates may continue for a second year of intensive leadership training. Some of our recent core groups have been designed and led entirely by core graduates.

In 1975, Sage extended its range of clinical services and investigation when it began its institutional program. Since then, Sage staff have been conducting groups in various institutional settings around the San Francisco Bay Area including homes for the aged, nursing homes, rest homes, and convalescent hospitals. Many of the residents of these institutions are severely limited in their physical and psychosocial functioning due to sickness, intense depression, and senility.

Sage institutional groups meet twice each week throughout the year and are composed of ten to twenty participants and two or more staff leaders. The program has been attempting to explore a variety of methods and techniques for body/mind development and revitalization in order to discover what methods and practices effectively generate the most worthwhile changes in the lives of the residents in these institutions. Drawing upon a wide range of techniques, activities, and human com-

Ken Dychtwald

munication skills, Sage staff have met with a great deal of success as many of the participants seem to experience heightened awareness, improved mental acuity, improved social and psychophysical skills, and an enhanced appreciation for their own self-responsibility as a result of their Sage experience. Because of the depressing conditions that prevail in many institutions of this type, the Sage institutional program has received a great deal of support from senior residences, institutions, and hospitals throughout the country.

Since the work that is being carried out by Sage suggests a variety of ways in which a humanistic self-development program can be effectively used to remedy the depression and bodymind decline of the later years, it is important that the techniques, instruments, and outcomes of this work be disseminated to the professional community at large. Preliminary research being carried out jointly by Morton Lieberman of the University of Chicago's Committee on Human Development and Dean Manheimer of the Institute for Research in Social Behavior in Berkeley, California has shown that the Sage approach in the core aroups has been significantly successful at lowering stress, heightening self-esteem, increasing coping skills, and several other key psychosocial variables.

When Sage began its work in 1974, its founders knew of few prople who were attempting to incorporate personal growth and holistic health methods and beliefs into their work with older people. Those who were experimenting with humanistically focused health, education, and recreation methods were doing so alone, usually with very little financial or psychological support and with minimal contact with others throughout the country who were involved with similar activities.

However, through outreach, training, and national development programs, Sage discovered that there was a growing number of people and institutions who were committed to many of the same innovative visions and practices. Although there had been a growing body of people and information that support a humanistic approach to gerontological services, programs, and research, there had not been a formal organization or network established to act as a clearinghouse and central resource agency for all of the shared ideas, techniques, materials, and experiences. As a result, many people and projects lacked support, stimulation, and relevant information-sharing.

In response to this situation, Sage gave birth to the Association for Humanistic Gerontology (A. H. G.). Founded by Sage co-director Ken Dychtwald in 1977, A. H. G. serves simultaneously as a professional association, an international resource-sharing network, and an information clearinghouse. After two years of operation,

A. H. G. has already attracted individual and organizational members from throughout the United States, Canada, South America, and several European countries. In this short time, A. H. G. has gathered and disseminated information on a wide assortment of innovative programs and creative ideas related to humanistic approaches to gerontology, psychology, and health care. To further coordinate information and provide local support, there are thirty regional A. H. G. coordinators located in key geographic locations.

A. H. G. 's first national conference was held in Berkeley, California in July, 1979. There was tremendous energy generated by the coming together of hundreds of people from hospitals and nursing homes, yoga centers and massage schools, the American Association for Retired Persons and the Gray Panthers.

The highlight of this exciting gathering was the sharing of information and ideas related to positively oriented programs for elders. Examples of programs of this type are the Senior Health Source in Albuquerque, New Mexico, which has developed a "health club" for elders, a day care center, and a hospice; The Nursing Home Residents' Advisory Council in Minneapolis, Minnesota, which trains elderly advocates in peer-counseling and helps nursing home residents take a more active role in shaping their lives; and the Seniors' Health Program of

Augustana Hospital in Chicago, Illinois, which offers workshops on topics such as medication safety, massage, and patients' rights to groups of elders at community centers.

Certainly no one method or technique will effectively remedy all of the problems of our older population. Yet it becomes increasingly urgent that just as lifestyles, healthstyles, and aging patterns have changed in the past few decades, so must the helping professions change to become more directly relevant to the unique needs and potentials of our continually expanding elder population. And if the trend toward disease prevention, health promotion, personal growth, and self-responsibility continues, it seems increasingly appropriate that more time, energy, and money be focused on pursuing those activities, programs, and methodologies that support a humanistically styled, holistic approach to mental and physical health for elders.

As architects of our own immediate and distant futures, we all need to explore creative ways to generate positive images of aging and full life development. This point was brought home to me vividly during a seminar on life design that I recently conducted at a local medical school. An elderly woman seated in the back of the room asked if she might make a point to the class. She stood up and stated that she was 78 years old and that when she was as young as we were, she had been very active in the social and political issues of her time. She explained that when she was in her 20's there was a great feeling of excitement and vision in America and, correspondingly, an enormous effort to "improve the world" and facilitate healthy and happy lifestyles for everyone.

This woman's face grew serious as she explained that in many ways the visions and dreams of her generation have been realized, though it took fifty years and two generations for the seeds they planted to take root and blossom. Now, however, she noted with sadness that there was something that she and yer young friends had neglected to consider when they were designing their "New Age": they had left out the elderly! Now that she had arrived at "old age," she unhappily realized that she had helped to shape a world in which she now does not fit.

Identifying and uprooting the ageism and negativity that pervade our culture will be a delicate and extremely arduous task — but a crucial one. Only if we can foster a new, more enlightened view of aging will we be able not only to improve our lives now but also to expand the possibilities that already exist in our collective future.

This is the task for Sage, for A. H. G., for all of us.

For more information, contact:

> Sage
> 114 Montecito Avenue
> Oakland, California 94610
>
> or
>
> Association for Humanistic Gerontology
> 1711 Solano Avenue
> Berkeley, California 94707

For additional reading, see:

Bodymind by Ken Dychtwald, Jove, 1978, $1.95. A synthesis of the human-potential movement that presents the techniques of Wilhelm Reich, Ida Rolf, Moshe Feldenkrois, Fritz Perls, Will Schultz, Alexander Lowen, and several types of yoga information in a manner understandable to the general public.

Lifetime — A New Image of Aging by Karen Preuss. Unity Press, Santa Cruz, California, 1978. $6.95. A wonderful photodocumentary of the Sage project.

Your Second Life by Gay Gaer Luce, Delacorte Press/Seymour Lawrence, New York, N. Y. 1979. A remarkable and practical book based on her work as a founder of Sage. It includes information and exercises related to breathing, dreaming, dying, meditating, relaxing, and exercising.

WE CAN DO IT!
AN INTERVIEW
WITH MAGGIE KUHN
by Robert J. Skeist, R. N.

Margaret E. (Maggie) Kuhn is co-founder and national spokesperson for the Gray Panthers, an activist organization of over 10,000 people of all ages committed to an end to discrimination on the basis of age, race or sex and to establishing social and economic justice.

She is the author of Get Out There and Do Something *(Friendship Press, 1972) and* Maggie Kuhn on Aging *(Westminster Press, 1977), and is the subject of the documentary film,* Maggie Kuhn: Wrinkled Radical. *Maggie lives in an intergenerational household in Philadelphia, where I interviewed her in 1979.*

RS: *The very existence of the Gray Panthers implies that there is a problem with the way old people are treated in our country. In describing this problem you have often used the term "ageism". What does this mean?*

MK: "Ageism" refers to the discrimination, segregation, and disabling of a group of people based on their chronological age. It results in a sense of alienation and powerlessness. It involves a set of prejudices that says that we old people, we elders, we survivors, are useless, senile, dumb, and ugly. We are supposed to all be crotchety and cranky, our brains shriveling up, and our sex organs withering away. All of that, of course, is nonsense.

The number of people 65 and older is steadily rising. Today we make up about 10% of the population, and in another 50 years we will be 20%. And what will happen with the old people? In some societies, like the Chinese or the Masai in Kenya, old people are deeply respected. But not here. America is caught up in the Detroit syndrome, and we scrap our old people like worn-out car hulks.

Most of the problems we face are reflections of the malfunctioning of society. There is a health care system based on profit — not on who needs care. There is a lack of decent housing. We are overdependent on the nuclear family as a source of love and support. Competition and loneliness are so widespread.

RS: *But many of those problems affect younger people, too.*

MK: Absolutely. And the Gray Panthers are not just a "silver-haired lobbying group," as the media sometimes portrays us. Our slogan is

"Age and Youth in Action." We see a connection between the problems of old people and racism, sexism, and issues of economic justice. Ageism, by the way, affects young people, too. A teenager might have the same problem an old person has in getting across an idea — we're not taken seriously.

RS: *I appreciate this chance to visit you in your home, amidst your books, plants, and cats. This is a pretty large house. Do you live here alone?*

MK: Oh, no! Nine people live in these two adjoining homes. You may have heard of one of them, Linda Horn, the nurse who co-authored the Gray Panther book on nursing homes. This is an intergenerational home. I'm the oldest at age 74. The youngest is 20.

RS: *Are you all related?*

MK: No, we're friends. We enjoy each other's company.

RS: *Isn't it unusual for old and young people to share a home?*

MK: Yes, unfortunately it is. There is a tendency to shut old people off from everyone else. It happens in nursing homes and in congregate living centers that the government subsidizes. Then there are the new developments like Sun City and Leisure World.

RS: *But I've spoken with some people in their 60's and 70's who say they prefer living in a building with others their age. They say young people make too much noise and don't share their interests.*

MK: Of course people should have that option. The problem is that too often there are no other choices. Most of us old folks still want to be part of this world. We need medical and housekeeping support so that more people can stay in their own homes. We need more intergenerational homes like this one, where old and young can benefit from each other. And we need to make neighborhoods safe, decent, and friendly — age-diverse communities where people help each other.

We elders can benefit from the energy and soul-searching of younger people. And we can give them our understanding, our experience in all kinds of work and social struggles. We can care for an educate the young and can monitor the courts. We have the time to speak out against dangerous nuclear energy, as the Gray Panthers spoke out against the war in Vietnam. Why should we cut ourselves off from life?

RS: *Maggie, I'm interested in your view on the lives of older women.*

MK: I suppose you know that we seem to last longer than men. Many women have lived mainly for their children and husbands and now are in a very tough situation. Their children are gone, their husbands are dead. Finances are very tight and the women don't feel they have a place in life. My friend Tish Sommers started a wonderful group called Displaced Home-makers to help the women build new lives. This grew into the Older Women's League, based in Oakland, California.

Sometimes a woman becomes a feminist late in life. In a women's organization she can find a support system, a new identity.

My own situation was quite different. I never married, I always worked hard at demanding jobs, and I've been a feminist for over 50 years. Way back in the 1920's I worked for the YWCA, conducting workers' education classes for young employed women.

RS: *What do you mean by "workers' education"?*

MK: At that time, women were not accepted into most trade unions. The YWCA was one of the few places where women could learn about work, solidarity, unions.

RS: *So many people I know who have reached age 50 or 60 worry a lot about illness and hospital bills. What actions have the Gray Panthers taken to improve health care for old people?*

MK: We've had some successful court cases. In Oregon in 1978, the Gray Panthers helped pass a ballot measure that allows people the freedom to buy dentures from either dentists or laboratory technicians called denturists. It's a good law. It guarantees that a dentist do a thorough mouth exam first. After that, the person can save hundreds of dollars by having a technician take the impression and do all the work on the false teeth.

We're looking for funds now to set up our "Healthy Block" programs. This will have two parts. First, we'll use space in a church to set up a wellness center. This will be a team effort. We already have medical and nursing schools interested in placing their students there. They will offer treatment, as well as a lot of screening and health education. Secondly, we will send people out into the community. They'll teach good health measures.

They'll also work for a safe and healthy environment. For example, here in Philadelphia we have 28,000 abandoned houses that are a terrible hazard. Community pressure can get them cleaned up.

If a project like this were started in Chicago, I think it could tie in well with your Seniors' Health Program at Augustana Hospital.

RS: *I think so, too. We place a lot of emphasis on patients' rights. Our nurses lead classes about heart conditions, exercise, massage and other health issues for groups of people over 60 years old.*

MK: I haven't heard of many programs like that, which is too bad. We need a lot more health education. People really can take responsibility for their own bodies, if the doctors and nurses explain things and show them some respect.

RS: *What do you think of groups like the Sage Project in California, that bring yoga, meditation and "human potential" techniques to old people?*

MK: They do excellent work, showing what should be obvious, that people can learn and grow at any age. The pleasures of all forms of exercise and spiritual growth should be available to old people. Why should they be just for the young middle class? But may I mention one hesitancy about those human potential groups? The inner journey is long, it perhaps endless, and individual growth alone doesn't change society. It doesn't change poverty and the social causes of alienation. "Holistic health" has to mean more than blending yoga with western medicine. It must include pressuring the corporations to stop polluting the environment, helping the unions get safe conditions at the workplace, dealing with the threat of nuclear annihilation, gaining full employment, and a host of other issues. The trick is to work together for these changes at the same time we care for ourselves and grow as individuals.

RS: *How does the health care system fit into your list of needed social changes?*

MK: First we need to agree that good health care is a basic right. No one argues that government should provide everyone with fire protection, police protection, or public schools. Health care is just as basic. This belief leads us to support the Congressman Ronald V. Dellums' bill to create a National Health Service (H. R. 2969).

RS: *I'm familiar with that bill. It embodies a lot of my beliefs about health care. The proposed National Health Service would provide high-quality health care to everyone, paid for by a progressive income tax. All health workers would be salaried, and poor and rural areas would be assured of adequate facilities and staff. There would be emphasis on safety at the workplace and in the environment and on education to help people maintain good health. Maggie, how do you respond to those who argue that such a National Health Service would be too expensive?*

An Interview with Maggie Kuhn

MK: I don't think it would be so expensive. As it stands now, we in the United States spend more on health care than any other country — about $800 per person per year. That's more than any western nation, even more than our defense budget, and it keeps going up. Right now there's lots of waste, such as neighboring hospitals each buying fantastically expensive equipment instead of sharing it. Some doctors charge outrageous fees, and others may perform unnecessary surgery because they get paid more for each operation. Then there are all those people hospitalized because home care is not taken seriously.

A lot of poor people go to hospitals for basic health services because there aren't good community health centers. Providing eye screenings, complete foot care, hearing aids, and other services not covered under Medicare should help older people stay independent and prevent some serious disabilities. As you mentioned, the National Health Service Act also calls for environmental controls and safer working conditions, which would cut down on diseases. All these measures will contribute to a more humane and reasonable health care system, and a less expensive one to boot.

RS: *After talking about such large issues, I'd like to bring our conversation back to a more personal level. You're a woman of 74 years. Several years* *after retirement, you're traveling around the country speaking and organizing, at a pace that would wear out most 20 year olds. How is your own health holding up?*

MK: Well, look at these hands — I do have arthritis. Plus some sort of throat ailment. I know what I should do — get extra rest and shut up for a change, but it seems hard to resist a good interview.

I've also had to deal with cancer. I had a serious carcinoma and was advised to have a radical hysterectomy. I was afraid, but my friends in the house helped give me the courage to face the operation. At surgery and afterward, it all went well. The doctor was surprised at how quickly an old lady like me could recover.

I had to recover quickly! After all, I have a lot left to do. We all do.

For further information on the Gray Panthers, or referral to the nearest local chapter, write or call:

Gray Panthers National Office
3635 Chestnut St.
Philadelphia, Pa. 19104
(215) 382-3300

This is also the address for the Gray Panthers Health Care Task Force and its committees on National Health Service, Health Legislation (for reform of Medicare, Medicaid, Medi-Gap insurance)

Health Education (for influencing the curricula and training of physicians, nurses, and other health workers), and Continuum of Care (for nursing home reform and expansion of home health services.)

Literature and other items available through the national office include:

Network, the Gray Panthers' bi-monthly newspaper; one year subscription	$5.00
Organization, libraries, and foreign subscription	$15.00
Gray Panthers' Manual for Organizing compiled by Harriet Perretz	$5.00
Citizens Action Guide for Nursing Home Reform; by Linda Horn and Elma Griesel	$4.50
Maggie Kuhn on Aging — A Dialog; edited by Dieter Hessel	$4.00
Gray Panther History	$1.00
Economic Study Guide	$1.25
Gray Panthers T-Shirts (Indicate gray or purple; small, medium or large)	$6.00
Poster — *Panthers on the Prowl*	$3.00
Buttons — *Gray Panthers: Age and Youth in Action*	$1.00

For further information related to the National Health Service, or referral to local groups working for its creation, contact the:

COALITION FOR A NATIONAL
HEALTH SERVICE
P. O. Box 6586
T Street Station
Washington D. C. 20009

Among the literature they offer is *Health Care for People — Not Profits* (free); reprints of the Congressional Digest of H. R. 2969 — U. S. Health Serivce Act (10¢); *What Price Health?* — a survey of the U. S. health scene by Joyce Goldstein ($1.50); *National Health Service: Lessons from Great Britain* by Meredith Turshen ($1.50); and *Women and a National Health Service* (free).